THE WELLNESS PUZZLE

*Creating optimal well-being,
one piece at a time*

ANDREW JOBLING

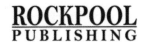

ROCKPOOL
PUBLISHING

A Rockpool book
Published by Rockpool Publishing
PO Box 252, Summer Hill, NSW 2130, Australia
www.rockpoolpublishing.com.au

First published in 2019
Copyright text © Andrew Jobling, 2019

ISBN 978-1-925682-81-6

A catalogue record for this book is available from the
National Library of Australia

Cover design by Farrah Careem
Cover images by Shutterstock
Editing by Lisa Macken
Internal images supplied by author
Typesetting and internal design by Sonya Murphy
Printed and bound in China
10 9 8 7 6 5 4 3 2 1

Contents

Foreword   v

Introduction   1

Earning the right: why would you listen to me?   5

A body out of balance   9

An evolution of wisdom   13

Putting together a puzzle   21

1. Find your purpose   27

2. Protect your mental and emotional spaces   43

3. Breathe easy   55

4. Something is in the water   65

5. The power of whole food   83

     Get the metabolic fire burning   93

     Cellular health: protect your unit of life   105

     Go with your gut   121

     Let food be thy medicine   133

     Nature provides everything we need   151

     All food is good!   173

6. Have faith in what you cannot see   193

7. Move your body

     One step at a time   213

     Stepping it up   231

Getting the complete picture   243

About the author   257

Foreword

'Let food be thy medicine, and medicine be thy food.' – Hippocrates

If you think this is just another health and wellness book, then think again. Despite every health guru endorsing another 'diet' that promises you'll be lean and happy by the last chapter, the reality is 95 per cent of diets fail: most people regain their lost weight within one to five years. Seventy-five per cent of women have unhealthy thoughts, feelings or behaviours related to food or their bodies. We currently live in a world with access to endless information and the opportunity to self-educate, yet find ourselves caught up with information overload, further increasing confusion about how to live happily and healthily.

As a qualified naturopath, fitness trainer and founder of Bec to Nature Naturopathy, I too have heard of the endless list of diets and exercise regimes on the market. I am passionate about educating my patients about how to return to basics by simply getting back to nature.

It is my hope and expectation that this book provides an effective learning experience and is action building for individuals desiring to improve their well-being *holistically* – piece by piece. This book assists in three key areas. First, it will equip you with the correct knowledge and provides easy, sustainable step-by step actions you can start today that will assist you with any barriers to health change, allowing you to be the best human being you can be. Second, it also strongly focuses on forming new healthy daily habits that can and will change your life forever. Third, it will challenge you to question yourself in areas of your life and health that you may have never considered vital for your physical, mental, emotional and spiritual well-being.

In closing, you will discover the honesty, wittiness and wisdom my friend Andrew has gained over many years of glorious mistakes and the various lessons learnt. It is the journey he has endured that has moulded him into the successful and educational best-selling author and key-note speaker he is today. Through this journey, he has impacted thousands of individuals to get more out of themselves and their lives through mentoring, speaking and writing. By the time you finish the last chapter I am confident you will be changing personal habits, which in turn will impact the people around you. It takes one individual to make a change that will then inspire others to evolve into their own best self. Be the change.

Bec Farah BHSc
Naturopath
Founder of Bec to Nature Naturopathy
www.bectonature.com.au
+61 451 969 909

Introduction

Get ready for the most amazing journey of your life.

This is not your normal wellness book. I'm not a guru, nor do I have all the answers. But guess what? You already *do* have the answers; you just may not know it! That's what this book is all about, to help you discover the answers to the optimal well-being you already have inside. I've been working in the wellness industry since the late 1980s as a personal trainer, speaker, mentor and now author. As you can imagine, I've worked with hundreds, maybe thousands, of people over that time. I can tell you, after all that time and with all my experience and knowledge, there is one and only one thing I am certain about: people will only do what they want to do!

All the knowledge, opportunity, motivation and inspiration in the world means absolutely nothing if you aren't compelled, don't know why and don't want to do what you need to do. You know what I'm talking about right now, don't you? There are more gyms, personal trainers, books, videos and online resources than we need, yet, as a world, we are unhealthier than ever before. Why? Only you can answer this question for yourself.

I don't know if you purchased this book, received it as a gift or are currently standing in a bookshop or reading this sample online and deciding if it's the right book for you to invest in. I do know that if you're reading, even just this introduction, you want to be leaner, fitter, more energised, healthier and happier in some way shape or form. Do you think this book might have the answers? Do you believe that there may be some secret solution within these pages to help you take your well-being to the next level? Do you need motivation or inspiration to do what you know – deep down – you should be doing?

Yes, I hope the answers you may be looking for are in this book. Yes, I believe there are some things I will cover about being optimally healthy you may be unaware of. Yes, it is my desire that you will feel motivated and inspired as you read these pages. The bottom line and the key question is: are you *ready now* to do what you need to do to take this information and apply it to your life and create optimal well-being? Make no mistake; you hold the power and the answers to take your well-being to any level you choose – *choose* being the operative word.

In this book I will talk in more detail about my hero, my mother Sue. She passed away at the end of 2004 after a 16-year journey with cancer. She was blasé and complacent about her health until she was diagnosed with terminal secondary cancer in her liver. Yes, I said secondary cancer. In other words, her initial diagnosis of breast cancer was not enough for her to take responsibility and ownership of her own well-being. Consequently, the secondary cancer appeared in her liver just 18 months after she was given the all-clear by doctors.

It was at this point, a critical crossroad in her life, Sue identified her 'why?' She made a decision to live and she started on a crusade to create optimal well-being for herself. This was a decision that turned a two- to three-year death sentence into a 15-year journey of joy, happiness, purpose and fulfilment. This was a period in her life, and mine, that inspires me every day. It is an incredibly moving and empowering story and I learned many, many valuable lessons through her example.

I hope through reading this book you can start to make some decisions before you are faced with a life-, career-, family- or personal-threatening crisis. I hope this book will inspire you to choose optimal well-being over just surviving and getting by. I hope it will empower you to take the simple steps I've outlined and make being the best you can be an exciting reality.

Just like a jigsaw puzzle, optimal well-being will happen one piece at a time. The key step in successfully completing a puzzle is that you have the picture on the front of the box. Similarly, the key to piecing together your wellness puzzle is that you have a clear, powerful and compelling picture of the person you want to be and the life you want to live.

Putting the pieces in place

At the end of each chapter there is a summary section just like this one. The idea is to take the information from the chapter to help you distil it down into a usable step-by-step action plan to move you from where you are today to a place of optimal well-being. Yes, I said *optimal well-being*: not just surviving, not just existing, not just being without sickness and not just getting through. I'm talking about living an incredible life of passion, purpose, energy, achievement, abundance and longevity. How does that sound?

There is also a 'Key questions and action steps' section that aims to help you not just learn something, not just understand something, not just agree with something, not just relate to something but to actually do something.

Welcome to my book. Enjoy my passion. Learn from my mistakes. Focus on yourself. Get ready for the most amazing journey of your life!

 Key questions and action steps

1. Are you ready to go?
2. Start reading.
3. Enjoy!

Earning the right: why would you listen to me?

This book is not an encyclopaedia of facts, research, science and comprehensive details; it will not give you all the answers. It's meant to provoke and challenge your current status quo.

You are a busy person; your time is valuable. You have many things that are important to you, and multiple priorities pulling you in different directions. You don't want to waste your time and energy on something that won't help you achieve the things you are aspiring to. You, therefore, need to ensure that whatever you invest time in will be worthwhile. Right?

I understand and respect that fact and so I am incredibly grateful that you have taken the time to even get to this very early stage in my book. It is my goal to make sure your time reading this book will not just be worth your while, not just positively impact your health, not just assist you in every area of your life, but also help you to make a positive difference in the lives of others.

I am so incredibly passionate about helping people be joyfully happy, optimally healthy and enthusiastically prosperous. It's been a purposeful pursuit of mine for almost 30 years. In fact, it has not waned over the years; if anything, it is stronger now than it has ever been.

I will talk more about the evolution of my thinking, the shaping of my beliefs and fuelling of this passion in more detail in the next few chapters. Right now, I need to make a confession: I'm not a doctor, I'm not a psychologist, I'm not a qualified nutritionist and I'm not highly academic. Actually, I'm an ex-footballer, a short-lived physical education teacher, a retired personal trainer and now a passionate author and speaker! I stumbled through four years of study to achieve my physical education degree but I do have almost 30 years of unique experiences and purposeful self-learning.

When I decided to write my first book, *Eat Chocolate, Drink Alcohol and Be Lean & Healthy*, I had to overcome a very strong and limiting belief. I believed that because I did not have the 'piece of paper', the 'qualification' or any conventional training, I was not worthy of writing a book about nutrition. Then I thought about it for a while. I realised that, at the time of starting to write that book, I already had almost 10 years' experience as a professional footballer, more than 15 years' experience as a fitness professional and personal trainer and thousands of hours of reading, listening and learning from some of the most qualified and credible people in the industry.

I recognised that what I actually had was life experience, personal experience and people experience and, at that point, I knew I was the best person to write that book. So I did, and today, some 15 years since publication, more than 35,000 sales later and after numerous testimonials of success, I know it was the right decision.

Soon after the book was published however, I wasn't feeling super confident about how it would go and what other more educated people would say about it. I remember in the early stages giving a copy to a dietician who read it and was far from positive. She told me, in no uncertain terms, that there were several things I'd written that weren't scientifically exact and that she could never recommend the book to her clients.

My confidence took a bit more of a beating!

Then with fear and apprehension I gave a copy to a highly qualified and globally successful nutritionist friend of mine. A few days later she sent me a message saying, 'I've read your book and have good news and bad news.' I was immediately worried. We spoke, and she explained that the good news was she thought the book was fantastic. Phew! The bad news she was referring to was her own bad news. I had written about the same things she wanted to write about in her own book – I felt amazing!

I knew then I had a message to share and I knew it would make a difference. I also knew that writing with exact detail and science wasn't and isn't my goal. My purpose was, instead, to write something that would simplify wellness, empower the reader and inspire people to take immediate action and create positive change in their lives.

So here I am now, another 15 years down the path, with a renewed vision and a determined focus to continue to push the message out about wellness. I'm 15 years older and hopefully 15 years wiser. After my thirty years in the industry, I definitely have a perspective I believe will enhance your life and consequently flow on to positively impact many people's lives for years and generations to come.

This book is not an encyclopaedia of facts, research, science and comprehensive details; it will not give you all the answers. Instead, it's meant to provoke and challenge your current status quo. Its intent is to encourage you to research areas that resonate with you the most. Its purpose is to help you identify areas that you need to change. My main motivation is that you will take charge and actually do something, right now, to create optimal wellness and complete your own optimal wellness puzzle.

Please enjoy my passion, understand my purpose and forgive my bad jokes. Read this book with yourself in mind. Read it with the only thought being how you can make a positive change in your well-being and your life. Read it, apply the information, and then through your actions inspire others to do the same.

You are meant to be lean, fit, healthy, happy, successful and prosperous. It is your birthright. Don't let failing health stop you. It's in your control so take action today!

Putting the pieces in place

What I've learned over the years and what I want you to know deep in your heart is this; when you know what you want to do, be or have and when you want it badly enough, you will always work out how to achieve it. The gaining of wisdom comes not through learning alone, it comes through continual motion. Through acting, falling, learning, picking yourself up and continuing to act you gain knowledge and wisdom. It comes with a deep desire for continual improvement and a decision to finish what you start. I urge you to make a decision now – when it comes to your wellness – to finish what you start!

 Key questions and action steps

1. Worry less about having all the details and knowledge and focus more on taking one small, simple action step towards better well-being, today.

2. One step at a time the answers, inspiration and results will come to you.

3. If you start reading this book, make a commitment to finish it. Deal?

A body out of balance

*You have the power and capacity to get your
mind and body back to optimal balance and
therefore create optimal wellness.*

What happened? You and I were born into an exciting world of opportunity
and possibility (and, by the way, it still is). You had goals, dreams, visions and
the expectation of a great life, didn't you? Hopefully you still do.

If you are pursuing them now and are on track for an amazing life, I say
good on you. If you're not, what happened to those goals and dreams? Have
you ended up spending most of your time doing something that you're really
not that passionate about? Are you in a place where you don't have enough
time with your family and friends? Is the time you actually do have with your
family and friends not the joyous time it should be because you feel flat, run
down and lethargic?

Are your energy levels not what you'd like them to be? Are you lethargic
instead of bouncing out of your skin? Have you lost the motivation to do the
things you need to do to be healthy? Are you doing what you said you would
never do: turning into your parents, falling into bad habits or giving up on

a better life? Do you speak to people, including yourself, in a way that you know is not how they, and you, deserve to be spoken to?

Have you discovered that extra spare tyre in exactly the place you don't want it? Are you suffering from allergies, skin issues and/or respiratory problems? Have you found yourself at the point where you are relying on medication to keep you functioning? Are you asking yourself how you ended up so out of balance?

These are questions that too many people are asking themselves every day. In fact, I have asked myself many of these questions over the years until I finally got to the place where I knew there was more available for me. There is for you, too. Are you ready for the answers?

My belief is that you were born to shine. You were put on this planet for a reason. You're here for a purpose: to do great things, to add value, to be successful and make a positive difference in the lives of others. Yes, I'm talking to you and about you – you are not just here to provide carbon dioxide for the plants!

You've been provided with an amazing body to help you achieve all these things. You're meant to be lean, fit and healthy. You're meant to be full of energy, and be enthusiastic and passionate about life. Your body has been equipped to keep you healthy and strong. It's been armed to fight off foreign objects, to keep you optimally well and to assist you in living a long, happy and healthy life.

This is how it's meant to be. This is why you were born and the natural way you were meant to live your life. This is a perfect scenario.

Well, we all know this is not a perfect world, don't we? So, what happened? Let me tell you: we were born into an imperfect world. We were born, and from the very moment we entered this world our bodies and minds were under attack from all angles and all sorts of unnatural and negative forces.

We were instantaneously impacted by pollution in the air we breathed and the water and food we consumed. We were immediately influenced by the fear, doubt and uncertainty of the world around us. We were automatically affected by the damage done to our environment over the years by generations of industrial and technological advancement. We were directly shaped by the attitudes, thinking and actions of those people closest to us. We were under attack from negative people, bad news and toxic thinking.

All of these influences impacted us: the way we think, the things we do, the fears that affect us, the confidence and the belief we have in ourselves. Stress was created through all of these negative forces, and that stress has and continues to have a physical impact on our mind and body. It has created an imbalance. It has caused dis-ease (the re-formatting of this word helps us to understand that 'disease' is simply a body lacking harmony). It has and is robbing you of the life you were destined to live.

Stress, anxiety, depression, inflammation, obesity, cancers, heart disease, diabetes, respiratory issues, skin disorders, lethargy, cravings, lack of motivation, poverty, anger, fear and any other negative situation you may be experiencing at the moment is just your body crying out to be loved and to be looked after. It's a body out of balance.

Are you ready for some good news? It can be changed! You have the power and capacity to get your mind and body back to optimal balance and therefore create optimal wellness. Are you ready to go on a journey that will change your life forever? Are you ready for optimal well-being? Are you ready to be lean, fit, healthy and happy? Are you ready to be the amazing person you were destined to be?

Do I hear 'yes'? Great: let's go!

Putting the pieces in place

The first step to regaining health and restoring balance is to understand that something needs to change, that you are ready and want something to change and that you are committed to making that change. If you're ready, this book will help you get back to the amazing 'YOU' you were meant to be. The only condition is that you are willing to take action on the ideas that are relevant for you.

Key questions and action steps

1. Is now the time for you to change your well-being and life?
2. Would you be willing to start today and take the first step?
3. You will be glad you did.

An evolution of wisdom

Knowledge can be gained in an instant, but wisdom will take a lifetime. Take the time to develop wisdom, and in the process you will find the answers that are currently eluding you.

Wow, was I clueless when I started in the health and fitness industry almost thirty years ago. I thought I knew everything, but I knew nothing! As I have recently entered my second half-century of life and am passionately and expectantly heading towards the magical 100-year mark, I can look back and see an incredible and transformational evolution of my thinking and attitudes towards optimal well-being.

It all started for me back in the 1980s as I was coming out of a seven-year professional football career and looking for my next career progression. I won't go into details of that football career in this book, as I have outlined all the gory details in a previous book. Needless to say, it was those seven years that dramatically influenced and shaped my young thinking, attitudes and actions as I started out in the health and fitness industry.

If you have had any experience in professional or high-level sport, then you'll understand what I mean when I tell you that the one word I resonate most with, as I think about that period of my life, is pain! Another word could be *torture*, maybe even *agony* would be apt. Regardless of the word, to date there is no other time in my life when I have been pushed so far outside my comfort zone so consistently and for so long.

Training was torturously painful. Being knocked around – and unconscious at times – by men many times bigger than me was brutally painful. Being abused and criticised by coaches was agonisingly painful. Being ridiculed, laughed at and insulted by spectators was embarrassingly painful. Yes, I believe the correct word I'm looking for is *pain*!

My professional football career was over when I was at the tender age of 24, and as I considered my next career step the fitness industry seemed to be a logical choice. I had a physical education degree and I loved sports, so working in gyms and becoming a personal trainer just seemed to be a natural transition. The biggest barrier to this career was my lack of common sense and knowledge when it came to helping the general population improve their health and fitness.

I had been indoctrinated for seven years with the attitude of 'no pain, no gain', 'go hard or go home' and 'all or nothing'. At no point in my seven years as a footballer, or even in my four years studying physical education, did I learn about the importance and impact of moderation, balance, recovery or good nutrition. What I learned was that I must train hard. Consequently, it was my firmly established belief that any goal was possible if you trained often enough, hard enough and for long enough.

As I started as a personal trainer, I had the faces, taunts and abuse of the cruel and heartless fitness trainers from my professional football days burned into my memory. I thought to myself: this is revenge time! I would train my clients hard and then they would pay me. It would be like a double bonus. So that's how I started my career. If my clients could walk out after a session I felt like I'd let them down, and if they vomited I thought it was their way of saying 'thank you'. Yep, I was clueless!

I'm sure you can imagine that my early days as a trainer were frustrating. My clients would regularly cancel, were often injured, weren't getting results and sometimes didn't even show up. I couldn't quite understand what was wrong with them all. I thought they were 'soft' and just needed to toughen up. After some self-reflection, however, I could see that the problem was looking back at me in the mirror. There was only one person common to each of these interactions and relationships, and that was me.

I started to see some flaws in my thinking and approach. I began to see some gaps in my knowledge. I became blatantly aware of my under-developed people skills. For some reason, yelling at them and demanding they toughen up just wasn't working. It was time to start learning about something that up until that point I hadn't considered, but now knew it was the missing link. It was nutrition.

I got hungry and pro-active for knowledge. I read books, went to seminars and workshops, watched videos and talked to experts, and over the next 12 months or so I got inspired. I tried things and I applied what I was learning to see how it actually worked in a practical sense. Me and several of my clients happily became my guinea pigs and over time everything started to fall into place, with no fatalities. It got to a point where I understood what had been missing for so long: the power of nutrition.

I read, understood and started to believe the great Greek philosopher Hippocrates, who said in the fourth century BCE: 'Let food be thy medicine and medicine be thy food.' I started to evangelistically share my newfound knowledge with everyone who would listen, and even those who wouldn't. I became one of those really annoying people who tried to change everyone, even those not wanting to change.

I started to think of ways to get my message out to a larger audience, even an audience who actually wanted to hear what I had to say. At that point, I made the decision to buy a café with the goal of providing great-tasting healthy food to educate, inspire and empower people to make better choices.

Then, as if working seven days per week in my personal training business and café wasn't enough, after two years I made the illogical decision to write a book. Why? I wanted to share the message. In 2002 the book was born, and in 2004 it was published.

I really thought I had all the answers. I believed that my knowledge of exercise and now nutrition meant I could help anyone and everyone. But something wasn't right. I would train my clients well; I would teach them about good nutrition. Why, then, were so many not getting results? I mean, they knew what to do, so, why weren't they doing it?

You know what I'm talking about, don't you? Let's face it, we're living in the technology and the information age: there is no shortage of data, education and inspiration about the steps to be lean, fit, healthy and happy. You really don't need to read this book to find the answers; you already know what you need to be doing. Everyone does. Do you believe me?

Well, let me ask you a few questions. Do you know you need to:

- eat a healthy breakfast every day?
- drink more water?
- eat more fruit and vegetables?
- eat more fish?
- eat less processed, packaged and takeaway foods?
- exercise regularly?
- sleep well?

If you didn't answer 'yes' to all of those questions, then I would be inclined to say liar, liar pants on fire! You know it, right? Therefore, the most important question is not about what you know, it's about what you are doing with what you know. That's a question only you can answer.

I began to realise that knowledge is not all that is required. If it was, we would all be lean, fit and healthy as we already know what we should be doing. Aha: another realisation came to me in my search for the answers to the wellness dilemma. It was this: the only reason why we wouldn't be doing what we know we should be doing is because we haven't yet connected those appropriate actions and our well-being with what is most important to us in our lives. Profound idea, right?

When I looked at the people who were doing the things they needed to do on a regular basis, they all had this one thing in common. When I observed these people doing uncomfortable things and creating good habits – whether they felt like it, wanted to or not – I could see the difference. It was focus. They had a bigger reason than just losing weight or being fit. They knew what was important to them and they understood that their well-being was a vital part of their bigger picture. They had good attitudes, they focused on their mindset and they made better decisions.

Okay, now I was certain I had all the answers, that the three keys were the right focus and mindset, regular exercise and good nutrition. Or so I thought … Why was it, then, there were and still are so many people who have good attitudes and positive focus, who eat well and exercise regularly but still get sick? I couldn't understand it, until my paradigm significantly shifted after reading a book called *The Magic is in the Extra Mile* by Larry Di Angi. The following three paragraphs changed my thinking forever:

A national news program conducted a study of fifty people who have lived over 100 years and still lead active, happy lives. The researchers specifically looked for similarities in diet, exercise, lifestyle and habits that could contribute to their longevity and quality of life. What they found was amazing.

We are becoming more and more aware of the great benefits of a healthy diet and exercise, and the researchers expected to find these factors to be the major contributors. Through an extensive interviewing process, the news team found that some of the participants in this study had what would be considered good diets. An equal number of people were not as healthy in their food choices. Exercise and other areas of lifestyle were also not found to be a common thread throughout the group.

However, two things were overwhelmingly consistent among over 90% of those studied. What were these consistent traits? Nine out of ten said that throughout their entire lives they awoke every morning with an *attitude of gratitude* for one more day of life and they *saw each day as a precious gift*. Secondly, nine out of ten stated that they felt that life was *too short to hold grudges or spend time complaining*, and *they forgave people quickly* and *refused to dwell on negative thoughts*. [My emphasis]

Aha: more answers! This made sense to me and it helped to explain the unexplainable, like why my Hungarian great-grandmother lived into her late nineties even though she smoked a carton of cigarettes every week, drank brandy and ate rich Hungarian food every day. She was smoked and pickled! Maybe, I initially thought, that's why she lived so long. Or, after my revelation, maybe it was because she loved her life, was grateful and saw each day as a precious gift.

It also cleared up that burning question about why so many relatively young people who eat well and exercise regularly, and who would be considered fit and healthy, get struck down with illness. It's the power of our mind: what we hold in our focus and the stress it can create in our body.

So, here I was with years of experience, wisdom, learning and ideas, believing I had all the answers and pieces to the wellness puzzle, but there was still more missing, I knew it! Even with all these qualities, attributes, attitudes and habits people were still getting sick. Why was it happening, and how could it be changed?

It's taken me 30 years and I know for a fact I still don't have all the answers, but I feel I am getting closer every day. What I want to offer you is seven pieces to this puzzle that will include; things that seem obvious to you, things you know, things you haven't even considered and things you will learn.

Optimal wellness will come by putting all the pieces into the puzzle because, as I'm sure you have experienced, there is nothing more frustrating and unsettling than an incomplete puzzle.

Putting the pieces in place

I guess the one thing I have learnt the most over almost 30 years as a wellness professional and more than 50 years on this planet is this: I will never and can never know it all, and I am always learning.

As you move forward through this book, I want to ask that you do so with an open mind. I would like to encourage you, no matter what you already know, to be ready, willing and excited to receive even one extra little gem that can make a difference for you. Decide to expect and believe that something you read in this book will be that one small piece, previously missing, that completes your wellness picture.

You see, knowledge can be gained in an instant, but wisdom will take a lifetime. The difference is that knowledge is what you think you know, and wisdom is what you know because you have lived it. Take the time to develop wisdom, and in the process you will find the answers that are currently eluding you.

 Key questions and action steps

1. Can you be honest with yourself and admit that you don't know it all? That takes courage to admit, so, well done.
2. Are you open to receive even one small piece that can totally change your whole deal?
3. Great! Get ready to put together the puzzle.

Putting together a puzzle

Complete your puzzle. Put all the pieces in place. Stop thinking, 'she'll be right, mate'. If you don't pay attention, she will most certainly NOT be right!

Have you ever put together a puzzle? I have to admit, I really don't have the patience. On the rare occasion I have started, committed myself to and actually finished a puzzle I felt very satisfied. Can you imagine, however, all the effort it takes to complete a puzzle, only to get to the very end and find a piece missing, the puzzle incomplete? It would be very unsettling and frustrating, as my father discovered.

My dad loved jigsaw puzzles. He was one of those unique people who had the patience and perseverance to spend hours sifting through thousands of pieces, sticking to the task and completing the picture. He would study the image on the front of the box, develop a strategy and get to work, one piece at a time.

Buying gifts for Dad on his birthdays and at Christmas was always easy; he got a jigsaw puzzle every single time. He had cupboards full of jigsaw puzzles of every type: beautiful scenery shots from all around the world, great masterpieces through history, classic cars, spectacular architecture and interesting people. After many years of buying him the 'standard' jigsaw puzzles, my brother and I – who were teenagers at the time – decided to try something a bit different and very cheeky.

We bought him a Playboy jigsaw puzzle – nude but tasteful. I have to admit when Dad unwrapped the package and looked at the picture on the box he was a bit excited, much to Mum's chagrin. He quickly set about clearing a space on the billiard table – which had been converted into his jigsaw puzzle workspace – and away he went. I had not seen him so enthusiastic about a puzzle, ever!

My brother and I had a quick conference and decided it would be an opportune time to play a little joke on Dad. When he had finished one of his sessions in the early stages of this puzzle, my brother and I got to work. I kept watch to make sure Dad was not in the vicinity and my brother fossicked through the pieces and carefully removed two of them. I'm pretty sure I don't need to tell you which two pieces we lifted!

Over the next few days Dad worked away diligently, excitedly and expectantly with his newest and most stimulating of puzzles. As he neared the end, and with only a few pieces left to complete the puzzle, we could see a disturbed look start to appear on his face. He knew something wasn't right, he knew something was missing. When there were finally no pieces left but the two most crucial pieces gone, he was distraught.

It was about that time my brother and I decided we best get out of there quickly. Dad stomped around the house yelling, 'Come here you kids and give me back my "bonza" bits!' He eventually caught us. We surrendered his bits, and with joy and satisfaction he slid them in place and completed his puzzle.

So, what's the point? None really, I just thought it was a fun story! Seriously, there are two points I want to highlight (pardon the pun). The first is that there is no way my dad, or anyone else for that matter, could complete a jigsaw puzzle unless they had the picture on the front of the box. Without a clear picture of what you want, most effort is futile. Second, unless all the pieces are included the puzzle is incomplete, and an incomplete puzzle is no puzzle at all – just as your wellness cannot be complete if each one of the pieces is not in place.

What about a television: do you know how it works? 'Who cares?' I imagine you saying, 'When is he going to get on with the steps to wellness?' Bear with me, because all these stories and analogies have a point that I hope will reinforce the message I'm trying to communicate.

This is my understanding of a TV: you sit on the couch, pick up the remote control, point it towards the television, press the power button and hey, presto, you have it! If you were to ask me how that actually happens, I can tell you with great confidence I have no idea. I'm guessing you are the same as me. It's just lucky there are some people in the world who understand the electronics and circuitry of your television.

I want you to try something if you're game. Go to your TV or computer monitor, open the back up and have a good look at the circuit board inside. You will see thousands of wires, connections, switches, plugs, dials and electronics. It's amazing to me how all of those components work together to bring a clear and sharp picture.

Okay, now pull out just one of the connections. Remove just one tiny little component out of the thousands that make up that circuit board. Will the TV or computer now work? Try it if you want to. The computer doesn't work, does it? If there is a picture on the monitor, it will be fuzzy or have lines through it. Simply because we disabled just one out of the thousands of components, the TV or computer stopped working. Hmmm …

Okay, so what has this got to do with wellness?

I'm about to share with you seven pieces of the wellness puzzle. Some of them you will be doing and some of them possibly not. If you want optimal health and, as you are reading this I assume you do, then if just one piece is missing the puzzle is incomplete. Leave out one piece of the puzzle and, just as the TV will not properly work, you cannot have the optimal health you want. Even worse is the potential long-term consequence of that missing piece. Just look around today and you will see millions of unhealthy, diseased and sick people who provide disturbing evidence of an incomplete wellness puzzle.

Are you with me?

It's my strongest encouragement that you read this book with an open mind and an honest evaluation of where you are at. Like me, you need to change some things if optimal well-being is your goal. Be honest with yourself, and let go of pride, stubbornness and outdated information. You will know what things relate to you. You will be aware of what pieces of the puzzle require your attention. Your intuition will cause a physical 'gut' reaction when you read something that you need to attend to. Please pay attention and take action.

If your TV doesn't work properly it's no big deal; you can live without it. In fact, my wife Laura and I lived with an annoying line running through our TV picture for many years. We don't watch TV that much so it didn't really bother us. It did, however, bother her brother, who often dog sits for us when we travel. We came home from a trip not long ago to find he had bought us a new TV with a crisp and clear picture. What a bonus!

If you lose the last piece of your jigsaw puzzle, it's annoying but not the end of the world. My dad was angry about his stolen bonza bits but he wasn't going to call search and rescue or do anything violent.

If, however, you disregard any part of your wellness then the cost may be one you don't want to pay. Why would you take that chance? Why wouldn't you do what you need to do to live your best life ever? Why not take some simple steps – right now – that will provide health, energy and the body you have always wanted? Go on, I dare you!

Putting the pieces in place

I think the message of this chapter is pretty self-explanatory, so I don't want to labour on it or insult your intelligence. I *do* want to make sure you take it seriously and don't just read it and say, 'that was interesting'.

Complete your puzzle. Put *all* the pieces in place. Stop thinking, 'she'll be right, mate'. If you don't pay attention, she will most certainly NOT be right! Please don't run the gauntlet with your health; there is too much to lose.

Here are the seven pieces of the wellness puzzle I will be covering:

- Puzzle Piece One: Find your purpose
- Puzzle Piece Two: Protect your mental and emotional spaces
- Puzzle Piece Three: Breathe easy
- Puzzle Piece Four: Something is in the water
- Puzzle Piece Five: The power of whole food
- Puzzle Piece Six: Have faith in what you cannot see
- Puzzle Piece Seven: Move your body

 ## Key questions and action steps

1. Stand up, shake yourself out and get ready to create optimal well-being.
2. Read forth and be happy, healthy and prosperous.

Find your purpose

Unless we identify our purpose and stay deliberately focused on it every day, the negative forces of life will take hold and push us down a path we don't want to go, but one we will eventually accept.

Imagine receiving 1,000 pieces of a jigsaw puzzle in a plastic bag: no box, and no picture of what the puzzle is meant to create. How would you go? There may be a marginal chance you could put it together but, if you are anything like me, you'd give up way before that could be a possibility. Honestly, without a clear picture the task of putting together a large jigsaw puzzle is almost a futile one – just as success in life and optimal well-being will be pointless without a clear picture of what you're working towards. You must have a clear and powerful purpose in life.

My tertiary education was something I had to do. At the time I was told I needed to make a decision about the path my career and life would take; I was a clueless 16 year old who could only see, think about and dream of a successful professional football career. When my parents told me to choose a course, they suggested a commerce, science or economics degree in order for me to keep my options open. My response was: 'Why would I want to do that? I'm going to be a professional footballer.' While I did eventually agree I should get a tertiary education, I didn't over-think it and I chose physical education. Why? Because it sounded like the closest thing to sport to me.

After somehow successfully fumbling my way through this four-year degree I accidentally became a school teacher. Why accidentally? Because when I chose the degree, so indifferent was I about it I didn't even know it was a teaching degree until the third year when I was told to arrange teaching rounds. So, at the age of 22 I started teaching physical education and mathematics to teenagers. It wasn't a passion, it wasn't my purpose and it certainly wasn't fun. In fact, it was simply something I had to do to earn money.

When my alarm went off, all I felt was anxiety. I would hit the snooze button as often as possible until I had no other choice but to drag myself out of bed and transition out of my dream time into my nightmare. I just didn't enjoy teaching teenagers who were there because they had to be, not because they wanted to be. I hated trying to force them to listen to me. I despised the discipline side of the job. I just felt sick to my stomach from the time I got up to the time I went to bed. I was thinking, 'This can't be good for me.'

I became a cranky and impatient person and often not fun to be around. Up until that time I had been a fun-loving, even slightly crazy kid, but I had changed. This job I was forcing myself to endure was changing my personality, and not for the better. I was drinking more than I should have because I needed to do something to dull the pain. I was eating poorly and my motivation to exercise just wasn't there any more. My energy levels were non-existent and my health was suffering. I had no passion and no purpose.

It finally got to the point where I could no longer force myself to accept this stressful scenario. I didn't enjoy my life, I didn't like the person I had become, and I certainly wasn't excited about my underwhelming income. I decided to quit teaching and move into the health and fitness industry.

I had dabbled over the previous year or so and worked a couple of evenings per week, after my teaching day was complete, in a gym. I really enjoyed it, so I thought this was the answer to my full-time career puzzle. I was wrong! I resigned from my teaching job and started working full time in the gym, where I lasted less than six months. I loved the job, but I couldn't relate to my boss. He was negative and critical, he was a bully and, to me, he was toxic!

I started to experience the same feelings of anxiety I had as a teacher. What was even worse was that I had taken a pay cut and so, in addition to having to endure a bully for a boss, I was now making even less money. This was another source of my stress. It didn't take me long to learn the lesson this time, and I discovered something about myself: I will not accept doing something I do not love. This boss made a critical and sarcastic comment to me one day that was the straw that broke the camel's back. It was the last insult I was prepared to take from him. I walked up to him, removed my staff shirt, handed it to him and told him exactly what he could do with his job!

I drove away that day feeling cold with no top on and uncertain about my next step, but relieved to be free from that toxic and unhealthy environment. I was excited about what my next step might be, and with that I made a few calls and soon I had another job in another gym. Not long after that I launched my personal training career.

Here is absolute evidence of the power of passion and a purpose. I went from working 8 am to 4 pm with 12 weeks per year paid holidays as a teacher, which was stressful and crappy, to working 5 am to 9 pm with no paid holidays as a personal trainer and I loved it! I bounced out of bed at 5 am, then powered through the day until 9 pm and I could have kept going. Passion gave me energy to burn. My purpose was to help people create positive change with their health and well-being. I had found my place, I had discovered my passion and I was living my purpose … or so I thought.

What I love most about life is that it's always providing lessons. There are times it even contradicts centuries of so-called wisdom. It has been said, and often credited to Confucius although unsubstantiated, that if you 'do what you love, you'll never work a day in your life'. This needs to have one small disclaimer added: 'unless you're doing it for money'. I can tell you that for the first few years of my personal training career I agreed with the statement: I truly loved it and thought I could do it forever.

However, after 15 years of getting up at 5 am and working 12 to 15 hours per day, six and sometimes seven days per week, things changed. What started out as a passion and purpose was, over time, reduced to a painful chore that had to be done to earn an income to pay for a lifestyle I had become accustomed to. Every dollar I earned was reliant on me getting up and being at work whether I felt like it or not, was healthy or not, enjoyed it or not. If I chose not to work or I couldn't work, I did not make one dollar.

I felt that stress and anxiety returning. I dreaded going to bed at night because I knew that in just a few short hours I would be forced to get up again to put up with many stinky and complaining clients whom I had to painfully convince to do things to look after their own well-being. I have to say here, just in case an ex-client of mine is reading this, I had many clients I loved training; they were committed to their own health and well-being and were a pleasure to work with. These people were just few and far between.

The biggest problem I was facing was that I was not looking after my own well-being. I was tired, run down, stressed, over-training and eating poorly and I'd lost my vision and purpose. I could see no light at the end of a long and dark tunnel. My attitude started to disintegrate and, again, I knew things had to change. But how?

I was doing what I knew to do: work hard. I had been taught my whole life that if I worked hard everything would be okay. That's just another piece of faulty wisdom, so I started learning and challenging myself to find the answers. I knew I needed to change my approach to health and fitness, so I studied nutrition and learned all I could. I knew I needed to improve my financial literacy so I read a book called *Rich Dad, Poor Dad* by Robert Kiyosaki that changed my whole paradigm about making money.

I got inspired about good nutrition and made one of the most illogical decisions I had ever made, and I've made a few! I thought that if I bought a café and provided healthy food, inspiring information and convenience to the people it might change my situation. Again, I was wrong. I did purchase a café and, in addition to my personal training business, I ended up working even harder. I worked 12 to 15 hours per day, now seven days per week, to find myself two years later nearly $100,000 in debt!

Okay, that didn't work, so what's next? You see, I was always looking to live a life of passion and purpose. I was always looking for the next thing and deep down I knew that all the decisions I'd made and the lessons I'd learned were just leading me to the point where I would find my true purpose. Finally, I was right! At this time in my career I made probably the most illogical decision I have ever made, but it somehow turned out to be the right one.

It was certainly not a sensible decision; it was definitely not based on any logical analysis and, considering my life at that time, it was totally unreasonable. However, I went with my intuition anyway and I decided to write a book! Who knew that being an author, sharing my knowledge and helping other people write books and chase unlikely success would be the purpose I was looking for? Who could have believed that this was what would feed me and fuel me to bounce out of bed and power through the day with passion?

I published my first book in 2004 and writing books continues to inspire and excite me every day. I'm more focused than ever, more excited than ever and more deliberate about my life than ever before. I'm healthier than I've ever been. I have no stress, only passion and purpose. At 54 years young I'm leaner, fitter and happier than I've ever been. I exercise six days per week, I eat well, I sleep like a champion and I make great decisions because my vision is to be writing books, travelling the world with my wife Laura and inspiring others to chase their dreams until I'm well over 100 years old. I can't do any of that without taking care of my well-being, today.

That's the power of purpose and passion. It's the most important piece in this wellness puzzle because it gives inspiration to make all the other pieces work. When we find our passion and purpose, when we're excited about life and we want to live every second of life, we immediately stop negotiating the price for better health. When we find our reason 'why' we stop debating, putting off and procrastinating. Instead, we just automatically do what we need to do to be optimally healthy, and we do it so we can continue to live our long, happy, successful and purpose-driven life.

Some science

I'm currently reading a book called *The Answer: How to discover what you want from life then make it happen* by Allan and Barbara Pease. The book talks a lot about your reticular activating system. In an ex-footballer's layman terms, it means that once you give your attention to something you will attract more of the same. So, get this: I'm obviously writing this chapter about purpose and goals in life and, magically, as I'm reading this particular book, I get to a part titled 'Clearly defined goals and life expectancy'. As I read it, I knew beyond any shadow of a doubt it needs to be shared here.

The authors discuss the work of Patrick Hill, from Carleton University in Canada, and Nicholas Turiano, from the University of Rochester Medical Center. They analysed data from 6,000 participants who were part of the 'Midlife in the United States' study that followed the lives of the subjects for 14 years. They focused on the participants' goals in life and their sense of purpose.

During the follow-up period, 569 of the participants had died. It was found and reported by Hill and Turiano that those who died had fewer goals – if any – and a lower purpose in life than those who were still living. Overall, individuals who declared having goals and a greater purpose in life had a significantly lower mortality risk. This was true across all age groups.

The findings of the researchers show that having a direction in life and setting clear goals for what you want to achieve helps you live longer. The earlier you start this process, if you haven't already, of finding your purpose and setting goals in life, the earlier these protective and preventative effects will happen.

On the flip side, cardiologist, author and founder of Revitalize-U, Dr Cynthia Thaik, talks about how negative emotions such as anger, anxiety, bitterness and hatred can have a devastating impact on the immune system. She talks about research that shows even one five-minute episode of negative emotion is so stressful that it can impair the immune system for more than six hours. Yikes! I can only wonder what sort of damage I did to my immune system in those years when I was not on purpose and just tolerating stressful situations.

In another study in 2003, Dr Richard Davidson and colleagues at the University of Wisconsin-Madison investigated the impact of emotions on flu risk. They asked 52 participants to recall the best and the worst times of their lives while having a brain scan. Next, the volunteers were given a flu vaccine and had their flu antibody levels measured six months later. Those who experienced particularly intense negative emotions (according to their brain activity) had fewer antibodies. In fact, the subjects who felt the worst made 50 per cent fewer antibodies than those who were less upset by their painful memories.

There are even studies that support the idea our emotional state will significantly impact the condition, strength and health of our DNA. Yes, this means that while we may be genetically predisposed to certain conditions because of family history, we can change our DNA. In other words, we can change our genetic stars!

Stem cell biologist and best-selling author Bruce Lipton, PhD says: 'When we have negative emotions such as anger, anxiety and dislike or hate, or think negative thoughts such as "I hate school", "I don't like so and so" or "Who does he/she think he is?", we experience stress and our energy reserves are redirected.' This causes a portion of our energy reserves that otherwise would be put to work maintaining, repairing and regenerating our complex biological systems to instead confront the stresses these negative thoughts and feelings create.

'In contrast,' he continues, 'when we activate the power of our heart's commitment and intentionally have sincere feelings such as appreciation, care and love, we allow our heart's electrical energy to work for us. Consciously choosing a core heart feeling over a negative one means instead of the drain and damage stress causes to our bodies' systems, we are renewed mentally, physically and emotionally. The more we do this the better we're able to ward off stress and energy drains in the future. Heartfelt positive feelings fortify our energy systems and nourish the body at the cellular level.' In simple terms most people can relate to, what this means is that when we are having a bad day, going through a rough period such as dealing with the sickness of a loved one or coping with financial troubles, we can actually influence our bodies – all the way down to the cellular level – by intentionally thinking positive thoughts and focusing on positive emotions.

Researchers have gone so far as to show that physical aspects of DNA strands could be influenced by human intention. The article 'Modulation of DNA Conformation by Heart-focused Intention' (McCraty, Atkinson & Tomasino, Institute of HeartMath, 2003) describes experiments that achieved such results. For example, an individual holding three DNA samples was directed to generate *heart coherence* – a beneficial state of mental, emotional and physical balance and harmony – with the aid of a technique that utilises heart breathing and intentional positive emotions.

The individual succeeded, as instructed, to intentionally and simultaneously unwind two of the DNA samples to different extents and leave the third unchanged. 'The results provide experimental evidence to support the hypothesis that aspects of the DNA molecule can be altered through intentionality,' the researchers state. 'The data indicates that when individuals are in a heart-focused, loving state and in a more coherent mode of physiological functioning, they have a greater ability to alter the conformation of DNA. Individuals capable of generating high ratios of heart coherence were able to alter DNA conformation according to their intention. Control group participants showed low ratios of heart coherence and were unable to intentionally alter the conformation of DNA.'

My hero

I have one other story I want to share with you to add more evidence to this research and to illustrate this powerful piece of the wellness puzzle. This story is about my hero and the person who has inspired me the most, my mother, Sue.

I'm not going to tell her whole story because it's available for you to read in my book about Sue's journey. What I do want to tell you is that she, like many people, had a challenging upbringing. Sue was born in 1935 in a communist Eastern European country and had a Jewish heritage. This was just four years before the outbreak of the Second World War and the horrendous Nazi regime. Need I say more?

Her childhood was impacted by uncertain times, with parents who, although well meaning and loving, were ill-equipped to raise a child and, at the same time, cope with moving their family from Hungary to Australia just before the outbreak of the war. Her adolescence was taken from her as she had to be a second mother to her sister and brother, who were eight and ten years younger respectively. Her adulthood was defined by an impoverished self-esteem that she developed as a child and teen. Her need was to feel accepted through working to earn love, from her parents and then her work-obsessed husband and three cute but demanding children.

She developed habits that weren't conducive to optimal health. Her thinking and low self-esteem would regularly take her down a path of anxiety and stress. She started smoking at a young age, which became a daily addictive pattern for many years. Moderate alcohol consumption became an unhealthy crutch that helped her cope with feelings of poor self-image. From an Eastern European background, eating rich foods and lots of cream sauces was just the norm.

Looking back now, it was really no surprise that she was diagnosed with breast cancer at the age of 53, which is ironically my current age as I write this section of the book. However, at the time, everyone including my mother couldn't quite believe her bad fortune. So, after some adjustment time, surgery and strong medication she was given a clean bill of health and confirmation that the cancer was gone and shouldn't return.

Notice I said *shouldn't*? It *shouldn't* return if some changes were made. It *shouldn't* return if there was a shift in mindset, self-love and emotional responses. It *shouldn't* return if she gave up smoking, drinking and rich foods. It *shouldn't* return if she started to purify her environment. Did Sue do any of those things? No, she didn't. Absolutely nothing changed. She didn't address or even consider the reasons why the cancer was there in the first place. She, and we, just naively hoped and assumed everything would be okay. Just for the record, hoping and assuming are bad strategies!

Consequently and not surprisingly the cancer reared its ugly head again just eighteen months later. This time it was a secondary cancer in her liver; this time the prognosis was not as optimistic. This time her life expectancy, from that moment, was predicted by the educated experts to be two to three years. This time, however, my mother said enough is enough and decided to take control. What happened from this point in her life is why I wrote a book about her. It is why she is, and always will be, my greatest hero!

Sue set a goal to live. She made a decision to prove the educated experts wrong. She knew that, if she was to change her circumstances, she needed to identify her 'why?' In other words, she needed to find her purpose for living. It didn't take her long. Her purpose was her family: those living and those still to come. She had a burning desire to be with her family to love them and to be loved by them. The moment she gained this clarity is the instant her life changed for the better.

This clarity opened her eyes to her reality. She could immediately see why she was in the situation she was in. She knew that if things were to change and she was to live, it was up to her. She took 100 per cent responsibility for where she had landed and she understood that 100 per cent ownership was required for her to move to a happy and healthy place.

I immediately noticed a significant change in her attitude, energy and actions. She instantly seemed happier and, even though she was dealing with life-threatening cancer, she was increasingly optimistic and solution focused. I think we would all believe, agree and understand that being optimistic and solution focused are better choices than the alternative.

Sue started to make the changes she needed to make. She stopped negotiating the price, compromising on herself and blaming external factors. She let go of victim thinking and took positive, consistent and focused action. Was it easy? Absolutely not, but it didn't matter any more, because at that moment no price was too high to pay for her beating this disease.

After decades of trying, she finally gave up smoking. Was it easy? No way, but definitely worth it. She was able to give up drinking. Did she miss it? I believe she did, but being around for her grandchildren was more important. She changed her eating habits from rich, fatty, processed and unhealthy foods to lean, organic, healthy and life-giving foods. Did she initially prefer the taste of the rich foods? You bet she did, but she had found a purpose greater than taste – in fact, she very quickly preferred the taste of good health!

Sue started juicing, purifying her water and air, meditating and affirming. She started to mend important troubled relationships and end toxic ones. She stopped watching the news and started watching uplifting and positive programs. She started living her life: travelling, experiencing, experimenting and giving. She handled the treatments better, recovered from side effects quicker and became a stronger, more confident and resilient person.

None of these changes were easy for Sue, however, they became non-negotiable. She did whatever she had to do to get back the life that had been so seriously threatened. The result of this attitude, focus and action was that she turned a two- to three-year death sentence into an amazing journey of 16 years. While we lost her at the tender age of 69, the last 16 years of her life were lived with purpose, to the fullest and with absolute passion. My mother was living evidence of the following (which has been attributed to various authors): 'Life is not measured by the number of breaths we take, but by the moments that take our breath away.'

Find your purpose and, almost like magic, the answers to all of your questions and concerns will appear before you.

Putting the pieces in place

I think it's pretty obvious why finding your purpose is so critical. If you're still unsure, have a look at your own life and the lives of the people around you. You will see people who are simply existing. As kids, life was exciting, wasn't it? There were no boundaries or obstacles and everything was possible. We were excited about every day and the amazing things we would do, have and achieve. We were all born with this purpose and potential, but for many people the purpose was beaten out of them over the years by parents, teachers, friends, society, jobs, bullies, challenges and adversity and by life.

Unless we identify our purpose and stay deliberately focused on it every day, the negative forces of life will take hold and push us down a path we don't want to go, but one we will eventually accept. Don't let it happen. Stop now and make the changes you need to make to live an exciting, purpose-driven and passionate life.

As mentioned, studies have shown that positive and purpose-driven people have more energy, stronger DNA, healthy hormones released in their bodies and significantly less physical symptoms of stress. Furthermore, people with a purpose and goals in life know they need optimal well-being to achieve everything they want. Therefore, they naturally and automatically make better decisions about their health: they eat better, exercise regularly, get more quality rest and seem to naturally live life easier.

On the other hand, there are people who have no purpose who struggle to get out of bed and then drag themselves through a lacklustre and uninspiring day. They have higher levels of stress and anxiety and, as a result, their immune system is impacted and they suffer from the physical consequences.

They are more likely to put off exercise, cancel healthy appointments, drink alcohol, smoke cigarettes, eat poorly and have a much higher risk of obesity, depression and disease.

Find your purpose and everything will change in a heartbeat. Here is a simple example to help you understand how things can so quickly change. Let's say tomorrow morning you have a dentist appointment at 8 am to get root canal work done. It's going to be a costly, painful and horrendous three hours of torture. How are you feeling the night before: stressed; anxious; terrified? What about when your alarm goes off in the morning: are you bouncing out of bed, full of energy, singing 'Hi ho, hi ho, it's off to have teeth pulled I go'? Or are you tired, lethargic, fearful, hiding under the covers and hitting snooze until there is no other choice but to get up? I think we know the answer, don't we?

But wait; there's a change to your plans. The night before you're supposed to go to the dentist you discover a letter that had fallen down the back of the couch. Inquisitively you open it to find it contains the first prize of a raffle you entered months ago but forgot all about. It's two first-class air tickets to Hawaii for a two-week stay in six-star holiday accommodation. You look at the dates on the tickets and realise that they are for flights leaving tomorrow morning at 6 am! It's an opportunity not to be missed, so with mixed emotions you cancel your dentist appointment. Those emotions are the greatest joy and immense happiness!

Now you've got a new plan in the morning: get to the airport for your free first-class-all-expenses-paid holiday to Hawaii. How are you feeling the night before now: excited; overjoyed; ecstatic? To get your 6 am flight you need to be at the airport by 4 am so you get up at 3 am. Any issues? None whatsoever. You'll bounce out of bed, won't you? In fact, you probably won't even sleep all night because you are too excited.

Let's be honest here: you're probably not going to find a letter down the back of the couch containing two free first-class tickets to Hawaii. Even if you did, it's not going to happen every two weeks, is it? So you're going to have to find something else that will create that positive energy and feeling of excitement every day to make your life a joyful pleasure rather than a painful chore.

I was sitting in a seminar several years ago and the speaker described how he had been struggling to achieve things in his life. He was suffering from anxiety, stress, procrastination and lethargy. He explained how one day he sat and started to think about what an ideal day would look like for him, if time and money were of no consequence. He spent an hour or so detailing this ideal day, from the moment he got up to the moment he went to bed. When he'd done it, he was excited. From that moment, every decision he had to make was easier because it had to contribute to this ideal day.

With that in mind, I got to work on my own ideal day and this is what I came up with:

I wake up when I finish sleeping in my luxurious bed next to my beautiful wife Laura and look out over the amazing view from our bedroom: the Amalfi coast in Italy.

I get up and do some exercise. We have a healthy breakfast and then we go for a walk along the waterfront.

I then settle into my office (with the inspiring view) for a couple of hours to write my next best-selling book.

I take Laura to lunch and we go shopping – she can spend as much money as she likes!

When we get home we prepare for guests coming over – friends and family who have travelled from around the world to visit us.

Our long table on the balcony overlooking the brilliant vista is covered with a delicious spread of beautiful fresh food and drink.

We eat, drink, laugh, share and are merry. I go to bed full … full of great food, full of joy, full of love and full of life.

An ideal day!

What a difference this one exercise has made in my life. I've printed it off and added images, and it sits on the wall in my office. In fact, I'm looking at it right now. It's in my shower and on the back of the toilet door. I look at it and imagine it many times every day. Every day this vision energises me and fuels my purpose and drives my actions. I can see the inspiring view from my balcony. I can feel the warm Italian breeze on my face. I can feel Laura's soft hand in mine as we walk along the waterfront. I can smell the beautifully fresh and tasty Italian food. I can feel the immense joy and satisfaction of my achievements. I am energised and excited, as I know it will be achieved.

Key questions and action steps

Are you ready to take action, identify your purpose and fuel your passion? *This is important.* Please do these activities, as your health, well-being and life depend on it.

1. Take some time to sit and think about what or who is most important to you.

2. List in order of importance your top five values.

3. From today onwards, filter every decision you make through these values and let your intuition guide you to make better decisions.

4. Describe an ideal day for you, if you had all the time and all the money you needed and wanted.

5. Type it out, add images and stick it up around your home so that every day it is in your face. Does this day excite you?

6. In the next twelve months, what will you achieve that will be a stepping stone to you living your ideal day? Write this goal in the following format: 'It is [add date] and I feel [add the way you will feel when it is achieved] as I have easily [add the measurable and specific goal].' Read this every day!

7. Write a list of at least five emotionally charged and compelling reasons why you will do what it takes to achieve this goal.

8. Find a mentor and/or accountability partner to help keep you on track every day to move towards this ideal day.

9. Be driven by your purpose; read your ideal day, your goals, your reason every day. Stay focused on the amazing life you want to live and maintain daily action, and your mind and body will do what it needs to do to bring it into an exciting and joyful reality.

References

The Answer: How to discover what you want from life then make it happen, Allan Pease and Barbara Pease, Orion Publishing Co., 2017

'Toxic Emotions Can Lead to Serious Health Problems', Dr Cynthia Thaik, https://www.huffingtonpost.com/dr-cynthia-thaik/emotional-wellness_b_4612392.html

2

Protect your mental and emotional spaces

Make no mistake: what you have, the things you achieve,
the wellness you enjoy and life you live is controlled by your
association and input.

An old Indian Cherokee chief was teaching his grandson about life. 'A fight is going on inside me,' he said to the boy. 'It is a terrible fight and it is between two wolves. One is evil: he is anger, envy, sorrow, regret, greed, arrogance, self-pity, guilt, resentment, inferiority, lies, false pride, superiority and ego.' The chief continued, 'The other is good: he is joy, peace, love, hope, serenity, humility, kindness, benevolence, empathy, generosity, truth, compassion, and faith. The same fight is going on inside you, and inside every other person, too.'

The grandson thought about it for a minute and then, with a concerned look on his face, asked his grandfather, 'Which wolf will win?'

The old Cherokee simply replied, 'The one you feed.'

Did you know that your thoughts control your life and your well-being? The wolf the old Indian Cherokee was referring to is your own inner voice or self-talk. The *good wolf* provides the positive words we use and the *evil wolf* provides the negative words we use and, as the wise Indian says, the words we use most will determine our life.

'How does this happen?' I hear you ask. It's very simple: your thoughts will determine your emotions, your emotions will create a physical response in the body and dictate your actions, your actions will develop into habits, and your habits will create your destiny. This destiny will be good or bad, happy or sad, healthy or diseased, prosperous or poor, successful or regretful, grateful or bitter, all depending on your thoughts.

Think of your own life and any area you are currently proud of and excited about. You are proud because you have successfully achieved something, right? It started with a thought which got you excited. You then made a decision, developed a plan, took control of your actions and created success because of the positive habits you developed. Well done, take a bow; you were responsible for your success.

Now, think of an area of your life about which you are regretful and disappointed. You are regretful because you missed an opportunity, found yourself in an undesirable situation or gave up on something, right? It started with a thought that clearly led to doubt, fear or other negative emotion. The result of that negative emotion probably caused procrastination or poor judgement, and a continual starting and stopping of the project at hand. Without even knowing what was happening, you were creating a habit of giving up that led to your regret. Fear not; all can change for you if you take responsibility for changing and protecting your thoughts.

In these two scenarios, I haven't really discussed the physical response to emotions before any actions are taken. In the previous chapter I mentioned that negative emotions will shut down the body's immune system. They also increase blood pressure and blood sugar levels (I will talk about this in later chapters). All of these things will lead to undesirable dis-ease. Laughter and positive emotions will strengthen your DNA, improve your immune system and lead to the release of healthy hormones in your body. Can you see how important your thoughts are?

Two different thought processes resulted in two very different outcomes for my mother in her journey with cancer. The initial diagnosis of breast cancer presented her with circumstances she believed to be out of her control. The way she responded, however, was totally her choice. Unfortunately, she chose the thoughts of a victim, of the why me and it's not fair nature. These thoughts then led to an emotional response of anger, fear and helplessness. As a result of these feelings, Sue simply presented herself to the medical profession to fix her, but deep down she was not really expecting a positive outcome. She couldn't yet see her role and responsibility in the disease. She naively followed the medical advice and took no positive action to enhance her well-being. The outcome of her initial thought process, 18 months later, was a far more aggressive secondary cancer appearing in her liver.

After the diagnosis of the secondary cancer, Sue chose a very different thought process. She started to think about her role in the disease, and see that her habits had possibly contributed. She started to think that if her actions had resulted in the cancer, then she also had the power to create well-being for herself. This thought process, as I'm sure you understand, led to a very different emotional response: hope, determination, empowerment and, to an extent, excitement that she could control her outcome. The actions she implemented from these emotions and the habits she created resulted in a 16-year journey of wellness, joy, love and fulfilment.

Our thoughts are our greatest ally or our worst enemy. The wonderful news is that they are within our control. This chapter is entirely devoted to helping you change and protect your thoughts so they will result in the life, success, fulfilment and wellness you want, rather than pain, dis-ease and regret. How does that sound?

Choose your associations carefully

Inspirational speaker Charlie 'Tremendous' Jones said: 'You will be the same person in five years as you are today except for two things: the people you meet and the books you read.' Why did he say that? Because he understood the power of the mind: the impact of our thoughts and how easily influenced we can be.

Have you ever heard about the power of association? Did you know you will become like the people you associate with? The great motivational speaker Jim Rohn said: 'You are the average of the five people you spend the most time with.' That will either excite or depress you, but what I really want it to do is wake you up, shake you around and help you understand the impact of the people you associate most with.

Would you agree that you act, talk and think in a similar way to your parents, whether you like it or not? Have you ever heard someone say, 'As hard as I tried not to, I'm becoming like my mother/father.' Have you ever said it? Why does it happen so regularly? Simple: for the first 20 years or more of your life you learned values, attitudes, habits and beliefs from them, whether you knew about it, wanted to, liked it or not. It was the power of association.

If you hang around complainers, you will complain. When you spend most of your time around smokers, you will smoke. Through your association with unhealthy people you will compromise your health. On the other hand, when you choose to associate with successful, happy, healthy and encouraging people you will start to become like them.

Think about groups you've been associated with. If you want to be part of and stay connected to any group, you have to behave like them or you will be ostracised. If you don't want to behave that way, then you will leave and find a new group. Be very careful about the people you choose to spend much of your life with: look at them, their lives, their relationships, their financial situation, their values, their language and their well-being. Do you want the same for yourself and your family (or future family)? If you do, then you've found the right group. If you don't, get out of there fast!

I remember taking some pretty extreme actions when I first started to understand the power of association and the need to be careful with whom I spent my time. After deciding to protect myself and my attitude, if I was ever faced with someone who was negative in their approach, attitude or language I would just turn and walk away. People often asked me if I ever offended anyone by walking away. I would respond, 'Honestly, I don't know. I don't hang around long enough to find out.'

You see, I am and have always been heavily influenced by the opinions of other people. From a young age, with middle-child-attention-seeking syndrome, I've always wanted to be accepted and liked. If you're anything like me, you'll know how stressful it can be. As a teenager, I often acted against my better judgement and outside my values to fit in with the 'cool' crowd. Every time I did, I was emotionally, anxiously and intuitively aware that I was doing the wrong thing.

I still feel remorse and guilt about how we treated one of our teachers when I was 15 years old. I'll refer to him as Mr X to preserve his anonymity. He was not meant to be a teacher; he had trouble controlling the class and was a prime candidate for teen ridicule because of his bottle-thick glasses and bucked teeth. We made life for this poor man an absolute misery: we laughed at him, threw things at him, hid from him and did any other horrible thing you can imagine a group of stinky teenage boys would do.

I don't know why I kept doing it. Actually, I do know why: it was my own insecurity and need to fit in with the crowd that motivated me to act outside of my value system. I always felt bad after each class with Mr X because, as we left the room, I could see the pain, misery and torment in his eyes. Sadly, that wasn't enough to stop me from doing it again and again and again; I had spent too long trying to be liked and accepted. It was not good for me, my personality, my decisions or my well-being.

Ironically, and maybe even deservedly, I experienced exactly what Mr X experienced when I was a teacher for those few short and painful years. The universe was paying me back. I don't have bucked teeth or wear thick-lensed glasses, but I certainly did feel the brunt of teenage insecurity and torment. I could see first hand the power of association and peer group pressure and the impact it had on the behaviour of teenagers, and the results they achieved.

Have you ever experienced bullying of any sort? Have you ever been subjected to ongoing criticism, ridicule or small-thinking people? The tragedy is that often these are the people closest to us; I'm sure you know what I mean. Have you ever worked in a toxic environment? Have you ever acted outside of your value system and against your intuition to fit in with a certain group, team or association? Have you ever left a certain group of people or association feeling flat, discouraged, heavy and despondent? I think we have all experienced one or more of these situations.

How do you feel when you associate with these people: happy, excited, enthusiastic, energised, optimistic and hopeful? Ha! In fact, I'm guessing it's the exact opposite; you feel angry, anxious, apathetic, lethargic, pessimistic and discouraged. It's not good, is it? It saps your energy and steals your dreams of a better life. It creates internal unrest, anxiety and stress, which can lead to many related conditions and dis-eases. It impacts your choices and your actions and consequently the habits you develop. These negative habits will have a detrimental impact on your health, relationships, financial situation and, in fact, your entire life.

Can you see why the right association is so important? I was well into my thirties when I realised that if I stayed in my current association I would be stuck there forever and would never live the life I dreamed of. I'd had a great career as a personal trainer for more than 15 years and I'd worked with some amazing people, but I knew that many of those people did not have the same vision or dreams I had. I knew if I stayed in that situation, with those people, I would probably not expand and push myself to create the life I wanted. Instead, I would have settled for what I had.

Absorb what I'm about say very carefully. Read, re-read, practise and live this statement until it is part of your DNA: 'I never settle for anything less than amazing and I always strive to live the life I am destined to live. I am good enough, I am worthy and I associate only with people who lift me, strengthen me and encourage me to be better.'

It was at that time in my life I knew I had to find a new group to associate with. I knew I needed to find people who had a big vision for their own lives, who wanted more and would help lift, stretch and encourage me. So that's exactly what I did. I politely and deliberately let go of people who would not be a part of my big picture and I found people who would not only help me, but would encourage every one of my crazy ideas and pursuits. It has made all the difference in my world.

Since that time, over 15 years ago, I have published seven books, I've created multiple income streams, I'm blissfully retired from my personal training career, I've met and married the most amazing woman of my dreams, I travel regularly, I'm optimally healthy and I love every second of my life. 'All this from your associations?' I hear you ask. My answer is a resounding 'yes!'

I love the story of a wonderful married couple, Rowan and Leila. Leila decided she wanted to get healthy and lose some weight and so she started a wellness program. Rowan, being the supportive husband, decided he would do it with her to encourage her. Through his association with his wife, who was taking positive action to change her circumstances, Rowan jokes that he 'accidentally' lost 20 kilograms (44 pounds)! It was no accident; it was the power of positive association. Leila, by the way, lost 30 kilograms (66 pounds) and they both have maintained that wellness status for more than 10 years. Again, this scenario for Rowan and Leila is largely to do with the positive associations they have developed in their life.

Can I suggest you carefully assess the attitudes and behaviours of the people with whom you most associate? You are unknowingly allowing them to determine your life!

Watch your thoughts: they become your words

Through associating with the right people, I was influenced in the direction I wanted to head. During the early stages of trying to re-calibrate myself, my thinking and my attitudes I learned there were many other toxic influences that could pull me, drag me and coerce me down a negative path. When you finally see the light, the darkness is more obvious and noticeable. I was acutely mindful of a more negative society and I became disturbingly aware of a predominantly doom and gloom attitude. I started to become increasingly sensitive to the overwhelming barrage of bad news reported on television and radio and in newspapers.

I started to experience the fear, uncertainty and anxiety that came with bad news. The more I watched, listened and read, the more I started to worry about disease, crime, terrorism and the economy. The more I knew, the more fear started to grip me and the less risks I was taking. I became scared of things that were largely in my own mind and an incorrect pre-conceived consequence. I mean, let's face it: there is absolutely nothing you and I can do about terrorism, crime and the economy. I decided that knowing about it just to 'keep up on current affairs' is a waste of the mental and emotional space I could be devoting to positive things and improving my own life.

I knew I could control *my* health, *my* economy and *my* success, so that is exactly what I needed to focus on. I started to realise that just associating with positive people wasn't enough: I had to purify my entire mental space. So I made a decision. Is it one I think you need to make? I don't know; that's up to you to decide, and it depends on the life you want to live.

I did something that many people think was extreme, and still today I get accused of being naive, ignorant and out of touch. I didn't care what others said; I knew I had to protect myself, my attitude and my well-being. I stopped watching the news and current affairs programs; I stopped reading newspapers and magazines; I stopped listening to the radio. I started attending more positive, educational and inspirational seminars, workshops and conferences. I started reading only books that would teach, reprogram and affirm what I wanted. I listened to audios while I was driving and I turned my car into a place of amazing learning and positive change.

Effectively, what I did was brainwash myself. Many people talk about brainwashing in a negative sense, but if your brain is dirty it needs to be washed. We never question that dirty clothes need to be laundered, dirty hair needs to be washed or dirty carpet needs to be vacuumed. So why is brainwashing a bad thing, especially when our brains are so badly soiled by negative people, bad news, polluted thinking, fear and stress? I say wash your brain, and wash it well. Wash it daily and cleanse it with the things that will purify your thoughts, erase your fear and doubts and raise your belief.

Choose carefully your words: they determine your actions

I started becoming very aware of the words I used, because I knew they were a reflection of my thinking and that they would determine my future health, wealth and happiness. I started to notice negative statements and thoughts such as 'I'm too busy', 'it's too hard', 'I'm not good enough', 'no one will like it', 'I'm too tired' and so on. I started to understand that my words would dictate my choices, which would control my actions, which would establish my habits, which would govern my destiny. I knew I needed to change the words and change them fast.

The reading, listening and attending I began to undertake were having a positive impact, but I knew I needed to start a deliberate and regular habit of positive affirming statements. Every time a negative thought came into my mind, I captured it and questioned it.

When the thought 'I can't because I'm too busy' came into my head, I captured it and asked myself, 'Is that what I want?' Clearly the answer was 'no', so I thought about what I wanted: 'I easily prioritise the time to

_____ because it's important to me.' When I captured the thought 'I'm not good enough', I replaced it with 'I am good enough and I do what's required to get the result.' I continued this process until I'd captured all my negative thoughts and replaced them with positive and powerful affirming statements. From that time and every day since, I read those statements out aloud to myself as I look at my handsome face in the mirror!

By controlling my words and developing a daily habit of affirming these positive statements, I noticed how I started to feel more empowered, excited and in control. These thoughts and words were creating the positive emotions that were, and are still, responsible for the physical response in my body and the actions I would take as a result. It's amazing how my life started to dramatically change, in many ways, as a result of these changes.

Understand your actions: they develop your habits and create your destiny

As I mentioned, it wasn't long after I had started to immerse myself in this world of positivity that things started to dramatically change for me. As I listened to, read, watched and affirmed successful thoughts and ideas, I started taking positive actions and creating powerful habits that were attracting those things to me. Funny how that works! I randomly – or maybe not – met a guy some 15 years ago who opened doors, introduced me to people and led me to a space that transformed the direction of my life. Through creating the right associations, I was able to dig my way out of my circumstances and change my health, wealth and happiness. It will do the same for you.

Putting the pieces in place

Everything you and I need to do to be optimally lean, fit, healthy and happy is just a decision away. The decision you make will be the result of a thought. The thought that leads to this decision is largely influenced by the environment you are in and what you allow into your head. Make no mistake: what you have, the things you achieve, the wellness you enjoy and life you live is controlled by your environment. For your own sake, make sure it's a positive environment and that the right stuff is going in.

Researchers once placed five monkeys in a cage. The cage had a ladder in the middle and bananas sitting on top of it. Every time a monkey went up the ladder in pursuit of a banana the scientists soaked the rest of the monkeys with ice-cold water. After a period of this happening, each time a monkey went up the ladder to get the bananas the others would pull him off the ladder and beat him up. Consequently, after some time, no monkey dared go up the ladder irrespective of the temptation.

The researchers then decided to substitute one of the monkeys. The first thing the new monkey did was climb the ladder to get the bananas, and immediately the other monkeys pulled him down and beat him up. After several beatings the new monkey learned not to climb the ladder, even though he never knew why. A second monkey was substituted and the same thing occurred, and this time the first new monkey participated in the beating up of the second new monkey. The substitutions continued until what was left was a cage of five new monkeys that, although they had never received a cold soaking, would continue to beat up any monkey that attempted to climb the ladder.

If the monkeys could talk and we asked them why they continued to beat up any monkey that attempted to climb the ladder they would say, 'I don't know, it's just what we do around here.' What are you thinking, saying and doing that doesn't seem quite right, but is just the way you do things? Where did it start and why is it continuing? It's the power of association and the influence of the people you hang around with and the input you get on a regular basis.

If you want different results, change the input!

 ## Key questions and action steps

1. Think about where most of your input is coming from. Is it lifting, encouraging, strengthening and inspiring you and helping you grow?
2. If you continue to associate with the people you're currently hanging around, will you have the optimal wellness and amazing life you want?

3. Have the courage to step away from the people who are dragging you down and actively search for people, groups and associations that will lift, encourage and support you.

4. What are you watching, reading and listening to – is it helping or harming you? Be honest with yourself; it's your life!

5. If you're not already, would you be willing to watch less TV and spend more time with inspiring people, improving your health, attending seminars and becoming a more happy, healthy and successful person?

6. If you're not already, would you be willing to read at least 15 minutes per day of a positive, inspiring, personal growth book? There are some amazing books out there, just find one you like and read.

7. If you're not already, would you be willing to turn off the radio in the car for a period of time and listen to inspiring and encouraging audios? Why not turn your car into a place of not just transport, but learning and inspiration?

8. Write a list of all your fears, doubts and concerns about living a better life. Look at each one and ask yourself if it's what you want. Then write a list of statements that describe exactly what you want and read it out aloud to yourself every day.

9. Commit to this routine until it becomes a daily ritual and watch your life fly to a new level of success as a result.

3

Breathe easy

The more I focus on my breathing the more I'm aware of my congestion. The more I'm conscious of air going in and out of my nose and lungs the more I can detect dust, pollution and odours.

I think we can all agree on the importance of the first two pieces of the wellness puzzle: finding your purpose and protecting your mental and emotional space. As I have explained, our thoughts, attitudes and emotions control our actions, habits and outcomes regarding our well-being and in our life. While we are becoming more aware and conscious of these things, I believe there is one thing in particular we are not as conscious of or seldom think about and we rarely consider its impact on our physical well-being. It's something we do every second, 24 hours per day, seven days per week.

Chef, nutritionist, author and friend of mine Sherry Strong (https://www. returntofood.com) has developed a concept she calls the nature principle. According to Sherry – and I love the simplicity of this principle – nature provides the nutrients we need in the quantities we need to consume them. She says that the more readily available and easy to access nutrients are, the more we need to consume them.

We will unpack this principle in detail over the next few chapters, but for now I want to ask you to consider the one nutrient that is most abundant and easily accessible in nature. It is a nutrient that is all around us. It is a nutrient that we can't survive without for even a few minutes. It is a nutrient we consume 24 hours per day and seven days per week whether we are awake or asleep.

Rather than come out and tell you exactly what it is – which of course you've already guessed – I'm going to ask you to do a quick activity and mathematical calculation I know will surprise you, as it did me. Can you find a stopwatch or timer to measure a 60-second interval? In that time, I want you to count the number of times you breathe in and out. Don't speed up or slow down your rate of breathing for the sake of the activity; just breathe in your normal way.

Please do this activity now, before you continue reading.

How did you go? I just did it and completed eighteen breaths; I'm guessing you got somewhere in the vicinity of 14 to 20 breaths. Okay, let's do some mathematics. I completed 18 breaths in one minute, which is 1,080 in an hour and 25,920 breaths in one full day. That's not just one day; that's every day. On average, we breathe 500 millilitres (17 ounces) of air into our lungs with each breath, so that equates to 12,960 litres (438,230 fluid ounces) of air, on average, going into my lungs every single day. What was your number?

Have you ever considered the volume of air entering your lungs on a daily basis? Have you really stopped to think about how critical breathing is in your life? If you don't believe me, just hold your breath for a couple of minutes and you will know! Breathing deeply does a myriad of things, all of which enhance your experience of life. According to www.onepowerfulword.com, proper breathing:

- detoxifies and releases toxins
- releases tension
- relaxes the mind and body and brings clarity
- relieves emotional problems
- relieves pain
- massages your organs
- increases muscle
- strengthens the immune system
- improves posture
- improves the quality of the blood
- increases digestion and assimilation of food
- improves the nervous system
- strengthens the lungs
- makes the heart stronger
- assists in weight control
- boosts energy levels and improves stamina
- improves cellular regeneration
- elevates moods

Okay, maybe don't really hold your breath for a couple of minutes! We know we can't live without it, but the question I want you to ponder right now is: have you ever considered *what is in the air* you breathe into your body 20,000 to 28,000 times each and every day? Have you reflected on the impact it may be having on your well-being? If not, I would ask you to consider it now.

It has been shown that the air inside is up to five times more polluted than the air outside. On average, we spend 90 per cent of our time inside with the most polluted room in the house – the bedroom. When you think about this, it makes sense. When do most people who suffer from asthma, snoring, congestion, allergies, sneezing and coughing and other respiratory issues suffer the most? At night, right?

If you look at and think about the 18 benefits of breathing listed above, a large number of them become nullified due to the pollution and toxicity that we take into our body from the air we breathe. I could go through them one by one and discuss how the quality of the air you breathe diminishes or negates the benefit that breathing pure air will provide. I don't want to depress you so early in the book, so I'll focus on what we can do about it. How does that sound?

The realisation of the impact of the air we breathe on our bodies answered many questions for me such as why it is that so many people who eat well, exercise regularly and have positive attitudes still suffer from allergies, inflammation and other dis-ease? It's because of that thing we automatically do and have unconsciously done, all day and every day, from the second we were slapped on the butt as a newborn baby – that is, breathe.

The good news is that we don't have to think about breathing. I mean, isn't it lucky we don't have to think about it? If we had to consciously take each breath we wouldn't get much sleep; we'd be too worried about forgetting to breathe. The bad news is we rarely think about the impact of the air we are breathing, unless of course you have some type of respiratory condition or you are in an obviously polluted area. It's the subtle and insidious toxins in the air – the ones we are unaware of and breathe every day – that are doing most of the damage.

What are you really breathing?

Outside, car exhaust, smoke, gases, pollution and all the other fumes are quite obvious and easily detected. It is, however, those sneaky pollutants in your home and your office that are causing most of the issues. You and I see people who leave their home with surgical masks placed over their nose and mouth to stop some of the environmental toxins entering their bodies. I used to laugh at them for looking silly and being obsessively pedantic, but I don't think that way any more. The greatest tragedy, however, is that when they get home they may believe they're safe from the pollution, and they probably take their masks off. This is the time when the greatest precautions need to be taken.

The names of some of the airborne contaminants that are currently residing in your home and waiting to enter your body have more letters than this sentence and are harder to pronounce than otorhinolaryngologist (an eye, nose and throat doctor). Needless to say, they are far better off in a medical dictionary than in your body.

There are **allergens** such as smoke, dust, pet allergens and dust-mite faeces, just to name a few; more than 10 different types of **bacteria,** including *Corynebacterium diphtheriae* (I picked an easy one); 15 to 20 **fungal spores,** including *Cladosporium sphaerospermum*; multiple **viruses,** including influenza A, rubella, mumps and many others; dozens of **pollens** such as birch, cedar, pollen fragments, nettles; and dangerous **minerals** such as fine road dust, asbestos, radon decay products, formaldehyde, dioxins, dibenzofurans and ozone.

Depressed; nervous; holding your breath? All are possible options, just not very good long-term strategies! I don't want to be negative, but I do want to make you aware that every breath of air going into your lungs is taking with it a nice cocktail of some of the above contaminants. Do you honestly believe optimal wellness is possible – and that's what I'm talking about here – if you are breathing in 12,000 to 13,000 litres (405,000 to 440,000 ounces) of polluted air each day? Even if only 10 per cent of the air you take into your lungs was contaminated – and I'm sure it's way more – that's still 1,200 to 1,300 litres (40,000 to 44,000 ounces) every day.

The current statistics on people with allergies, asthma, respiratory issues and other related diseases are rampant in the 21st century. Why? That's the question we should all be asking. I don't buy the theory that we are born with allergies, that it is genetic or that it's just bad luck. It's not luck; it's largely the choices we make and the environment we are exposed to. I don't believe drugs are the answer to most issues. They are a quick fix bandage reaction that will perpetuate the condition and have serious side effects, and are absolutely *not* getting to the root cause.

I'm not a doctor, I'm not a scientist and I haven't done years of research and double-blinded studies, so disregard what I'm about to say if that's the evidence and credentials you need. I'm a passionate observer and I've been in the industry of wellness and prevention for almost 30 years, and there is just too much anecdotal evidence to ignore. The long-term solution lies not in treating the symptoms. I believe the answer is cutting off the toxins that cause the symptoms at the source.

The solution

If the cause of the allergies, asthma and illness you and your family are suffering is in the air, then wouldn't it be worth purifying that air to save your lungs, body and your health, not to mention your bank account? I'm not asthmatic, but I would bet that ongoing pharmaceuticals are an expense most families could do without.

Let's not get stressed or obsessed about this; let's get solution oriented. Let's control what we can control. What you can't control is the air outside, and the best you can do to counter that is wear a surgical mask. That's your choice. We can, however, control the air inside. Isn't that great news? It's especially good considering you spend 80 to 90 per cent of your time indoors and therefore you can purify 10,000 to 11,000 litres (340,000 to 370,000 fluid ounces) of the air you breathe every day.

Purify, purify, purify! Clean the air in your home and in your office. It's available, it's effective and it's worth it. There are several quality air purifiers, salt lamps and other purification options available on the market that will do exactly what I'm talking about, that is, purify the air that goes into your lungs. This is not an air purifier sales pitch; it is, however, a strong encouragement for you to make the investment now to significantly reduce the risk of a much greater cost should the pollution entering your lungs impact your health or that of your family.

My father-in-law, Laura's dad, is a classic and chronic snorer. I'm talking earth-shattering and glass-breaking snoring. He is one of the great wonders of the modern world because his snoring can be heard from the moon. Okay, so I exaggerated a little bit, but it used to be a serious problem. It impacted his sleep and it affected my mother-in-law's sleep, which in turn influenced the quality of their relationship. Do you live with a snorer, or are you a snorer? What causes snoring? If you could fix it overnight, would that be of interest?

We lent our air purifier to Laura's parents to trial for a couple of nights. After just one night Laura's mother rang to request that Laura come and get the 'stupid machine' and take it away. When Laura questioned her mother, the response she got was: 'I didn't sleep for one second. Your father did not make a sound all night and I had to keep checking to see if he was alive!' Needless to say, they purchased a purifier. Laura's mother got used to her husband not snoring and life has been great for both of them ever since.

This is not an isolated example; we have seen this time and time and time again. Overnight: snoring cured! In one night, the dust and other pollutants that were getting stuck in the nasal passage and causing that harmonic and reverberating sound were eliminated from the air. The source of the problem was removed and the issue was solved. No drugs. No violence. No stress.

I can give you dozens of examples of people with asthma and other respiratory issues who have experienced a significant improvement *overnight* by simply purifying the air in their homes and bedrooms. It's simple: remove the source of the problem, and the first step in finding a solution has been taken.

What about people who aren't snorers, don't suffer from respiratory issues or aren't affected by allergies or other common conditions? That's a great question and, in my opinion, it's an even greater reason to take measures to purify the air. Everything in life is cause and effect. The result you have or will have is the direct or indirect effect of the choices you make and actions you take. Are you feeling great at the moment? If so, why not do everything you can to stay that way? Why not pass on healthy habits and practices to your children and important people in your life to ensure they also stay healthy and happy?

It's a tragedy that so many people live by the old 'she'll-be-right' attitude when it comes to their health and well-being. They make ill-considered decisions that lead to questionable habits that often lead to conditions which they erroneously believe are the result of bad luck. It's not luck; it's poor judgement. The truth is that 'she most definitely won't be right' unless you take positive, pro-active and preventative measures now!

Remember, I'm talking about optimal wellness here. I'm not talking about merely surviving. I'm not talking about just getting through the day. I'm encouraging you to step above the pack and live a life of abundance that you are passionate about. I want to help you live to be 100 years old (if that's what you want) and have the same energy you had as a 20 year old. If you're interested in that – which I assume you are, or you would've given up reading this book a long time ago – understand it can't happen unless you control that substance that is entering and impacting your body 24/7. That is: air!

Putting the pieces in place

I don't think there is too much more to say here, is there? Having said that, I would like to talk about something I've recently undertaken. I started working with an amazing man who has been focusing on meditating, breathing and relaxation for more than 40 years. He is a wise, calming and inspiring man who is helping me get out of my busy head and into the joy, beauty and wonder of the present moment.

For the last couple of weeks (as I write this section of the book) I have been actively partaking in daily breathing and meditation practice. The primary focus of this practice is breathing. The more I focus on my breathing the more I'm aware of my congestion. The more I'm conscious of air going in and out of my nose and lungs the more I can detect dust, pollution and odours. In the last few weeks, the whole idea of air purification has been further stamped in my heart and soul as not just an interesting and compelling theory, but an absolute imperative.

I know that 97 per cent of the people who read this chapter will think it sounds like a good idea – something that should be considered – then do nothing about it. I hope you are a part of the three per cent who will do further research and take positive action to make sure the air – the most abundant and necessary nutrient entering your body every second of every day – is pure and able to do all the amazing things it's meant to do.

 Key questions and action steps

1. Are you interested in further research about air quality and the impact it's having on you and your family?
2. If so, do it!
3. Start to research different types of air purification units and trial as many as you can.
4. If you want more information or any help about finding a high-quality air purification unit, please contact me through the landing page: http://andrewjobling.com.au/books/wellness-puzzle/

4

Something is in the water

Water is a magical liquid. Water can give life,
protect life and enhance life. Drink enough of the right type
of water and experience how it will help you live the life
of optimal wellness for which you are striving.

Let's get back to Sherry Strong's nature principle – it's a good one! The most abundant and readily available (although polluted) nutrient on the planet and the one we need to consume most is air. The second most abundant and readily available nutrient on the planet and one we rely on the second most is – you guessed it – water. But please don't try to drink 13,000 litres per day.

I once set myself the crazy task of drinking 10 litres (338 fluid ounces) in one day. Why? I can't really say, except that I was, am and always will be an attention-seeking middle child. I was personal training at the time, and me and another trainer challenged each other to this momentous task. We started early in the day, smashed down a couple of litres quickly and thought it would be a piece of cake. We were wrong; horribly wrong!

Halfway through the day, about five litres and ten toilet visits into this journey, I started to slow down, but I was determined so I kept going. With every mouthful after that point it felt like water was leaking out my ears. I sipped, gulped, slurped, burped, gurgled and bubbled my way to nine litres of water for the day. I was officially done. I could not put one more drop of liquid into my waterlogged body. For the next few days I felt terrible, so if you're asking yourself, 'can I drink too much water?' the answer is a categorical YES!

Having said that, you know you need to probably drink more water than you're drinking now, don't you? Do you know how much you should be drinking? Do you know how much you currently are drinking? Could you, for the sake of your health and well-being, develop a strategy over the next month or so to gradually increase your water intake?

This chapter is not about sharing all the reasons why you need to drink water. I don't want to bore you, insult your intelligence or tell you what to do. What I will do is steal some of my own material to give you a quick overview of some interesting information. The following facts and statistics are from one of my previous books; I have given myself written permission to use it!

The reality is that there isn't one bodily function that does not depend on water. In fact, 60 to 70 per cent of the human body is water. Have a think about how your body would be without it – not much more than a pile of dust.

The following table indicates what percentage of various body parts is water:

Teeth	10%
Bones	13%
Cartilage	55%
Red blood corpuscles	69%
Liver	72%
Muscle tissue	75%
Spleen	76%

Lungs	80%
Brain	81%
Bile	86%
Plasma	90%
Blood (all components)	91%
Lymph	94%
Gastric juice	96%
Saliva	96%

Is it time for a drink?

Some of the more important functions of water are as follows:

- Water supports and aids every process, from digestion and absorption of food and nutrients to utilisation and excretion. From the moment food enters your mouth, every process to transform it from its original state to blood, bone, muscle and tissues relies on water.

- As we know, food is broken down into the nutrients necessary for life through processes requiring water. Those nutrients are then held in solution and transported to the various body parts in water.

- Water holds the wastes and toxins it collects from the cells and carries them to the appropriate organs for elimination.

- Water is a vital ingredient of all cells and tissues and of all body fluids. For example, saliva, gastric juices, blood and so on are all over ninety per cent water.

- Water keeps various mucous membranes of the body soft and lubricated and prevents rubbing or friction between tissue surfaces. This enhances the body's ability to move and an organ's ability to function and the suppleness of muscles.

- Water is the chief agent in regulating body temperature. This is vital, as an internal temperature change of only a few degrees can be life threatening and result in death.

I once heard a really simple way to calculate the minimum amount of water you need to consume for good health. How accurate it is I don't know, but it's been very effective for me and many people I've worked with. If you take your weight in kilograms and divide it by 30 (or your weight in pounds and divide it by 66) you will arrive at the answer.

For example, if I weigh 90 kilograms (200 pounds), then I need to consume at least three litres of water per day. This minimum number will need to increase if you frequently lose water through sweat, which happens from exercising, having an active profession or living in a humid climate. You will also need to drink more water if you regularly consume substances that dehydrate the body such as caffeine, alcohol, soft drinks, processed foods and tap water. Yes, I said tap water! The chemical and toxic cocktail that is in tap water all around the world requires that your body work harder to eliminate it. Among other things, this requires water – pure water!

Apart from not drinking enough water, which is an issue for most people, what's in the water we do drink (like our air) is causing much of the imbalance and dis-ease I've already spoken about. Remember, water is the second most readily available and abundant nutrient on the planet, and the second most needed and consumed nutrient we put in our body. Again, I ask the question: do you know what's in the water you are drinking?

We tend to consume our water in different ways and from different sources. Let me first inform those of you who are kidding yourselves that the water in coffee and caffeinated drinks, juices, soft drinks and alcohol doesn't count. In fact, those drinks will add toxins that will start to create imbalance, dehydrate you and increase the volume of water you actually need to drink for the day. Devastating, but true!

One simple and healthy strategy to increase your intake without drinking more water is to eat foods with high water content. I don't mean icy poles, popsicles, soft serve or slurpees! I do mean fruits, vegetables and plant-based foods but, of course, you already knew that, didn't you?

So again, the main aim of this chapter is not to bore you with stuff you've heard about time and time again. This chapter is to help you understand and be clearly aware that, as much a part of the solution to good health water may be, it can also be a major part of the problem. Let me explain this further by telling you the story of Ronnie the raindrop and his friends Ralph, Rex, Rudolph, Rachel, Roxie and Renata.

Ronnie the raindrop

Ronnie and his friends lived blissfully and comfortably in a beautiful soft and fluffy cloud floating majestically many kilometres above the earth. The only thing that often spoiled their existence was a toxic smell that wafted through the cloud from passing flying machines and the smoke rising from the earth and cities below. Ronnie wasn't sure, but somehow he could feel those toxins infiltrating his small and fragile body.

As more raindrops moved into the cloud it became busier and more crowded, and the weight of Ronnie and his increasing number of friends started to take its toll on the cloud. In the confined spaces the raindrops started to annoy each other, argue and even start pushing and shoving. After a short time, some of the raindrops decided to leave. They said goodbye to their friends and jumped.

One by one, Ronnie's friends leapt out of the cloud and started falling towards the earth. Not wanting to miss out, Ronnie closed his eyes, held his breath and took that leap of faith. Falling through the air was initially terrifying for him, but soon became exhilarating. He loved the freedom he felt as he accelerated towards the ground with the wind in his face.

He did notice, however, that the closer he got to the ground, the toxic fumes he could smell in the cloud were getting stronger and the air was getting thicker. Just before he landed, he caught a glimpse of himself in the reflection of another raindrop and his face was dusty, dirty and brown. Finally, he landed with a splash in a large reservoir of water made up of all his friends from his cloud and raindrops from many other clouds. He had fun finding and re-uniting with Ralph, Rex, Rudolph, Rachel, Roxie and Renata.

Life in the reservoir wasn't the same as life in the cloud. It was crowded and stressful and many foreign objects were entering the body of water and impacting all the little raindrops. Large animals were swimming through the water with dirty and muddy feet and fur. Those same animals thought it was a great place to dump their stinky waste products. Many animals were becoming lifeless in the water and decomposing, leaving their bacteria and germs to contaminate Ronnie and his friends. There were even funny-looking two-legged human animals throwing their rubbish into Ronnie's home. Every day he could feel himself getting more and more contaminated by all the foreign objects.

One day, as he was floating around trying to survive, he could feel himself being pulled. He tried to resist the force but, alas, he was too small and weak. He found himself being sucked into a large round opening that lead to a long dark tunnel. As he entered the tunnel, he and his friends started moving at a frantic pace for what seemed to be an eternity. He was terrified, but finally noticed he was rapidly approaching a light at the end of the tunnel. He flew out of it and landed in another pool of water.

There was a moment of relief, but it was short lived as Ronnie then felt himself being covered with a chemical spray. Initially, he felt it cleansing him from all the dirt, bacteria, germs and contamination that had enveloped him in the reservoir, but that relief soon turned to distress. He started coughing and wheezing and had as much trouble breathing as you could imagine a raindrop would.

Ronnie and friends were out of control as these chemicals attacked their small, vulnerable bodies and then, again, they were sucked forcefully into another dark tunnel. This one was pitch black. It was long, it was dark, it was smelly and there seemed no end in sight. The seconds rolled into minutes, the minutes flowed into hours and Ronnie and his raindrop friends were pulled helplessly along this seemingly endless tunnel of terror.

Dead and dying animals, animal faeces, mould, rust and all manner of disgusting things flowed with them, bumped into them and passed by them on the journey to 'who knows where'. With each metre they travelled, they could feel all the chemicals, bacteria, viruses, pollutants and toxins attack them and being absorbed into their little bodies.

Finally, after many hours, maybe even days, Ronnie saw a light at the end of this tunnel and he felt himself being pulled up towards the light. The closer he got to the light, the tighter the pipes became and the more they began to twist and turn. The pressure was building, his speed was increasing and he screamed as he was shot out of a tap at breakneck speed and into a small clear container.

Now he was floating in this new small glass vessel with a few of his friends. He felt dirty, polluted and violated, and as he looked up he could see that he was getting closer and closer to the open mouth of a child. He knew he was toxic and dangerous and could hurt that child. He started yelling as loud as he could to stop the child from swallowing him. It was all to no avail as raindrops don't have vocal chords. The child couldn't hear him and continued to consume Ronnie, his friends and all of the disgusting toxic chemicals and pollutants that were with them.

And everyone lived toxically ever after!

I think these days most people are well aware of the fact that drinking water straight out of a tap is not the best option. Otherwise, why would we be spending such a ridiculous amount of money on bottled water? I'll talk more about bottled water shortly. There are still people who may be unsure about why drinking tap water is not the best option. I live in Melbourne, Australia and continually hear that Melbourne tap water is the best tap water in the world. That may be so, but compared to what? It's possibly better to drink petrol than hydrochloric acid, but not for one second does that mean you should consider drinking petrol.

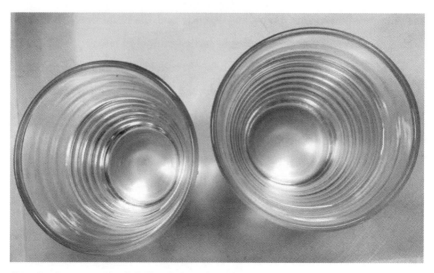

Discolored tap water in right hand glass, clear, pure water in left hand glass.

One of the many issues that impacted Ronnie the raindrop and his friends was the chlorine and other chemicals added to the water at the treatment plant as they began their journey from the reservoir through many hundreds of kilometres of pipes as they flow towards your tap. The idea of the chlorine is a noble one. It's added to kill the viruses and bacteria that can have a dramatic and immediate negative impact on our health. The problem is that chlorine is a poison that kills living viruses and bacteria. I'll say that again: chlorine is a poison that kills living things.

Any time you walk into an indoor swimming pool, the thing you will notice first is the overpowering smell of chlorine, right? Chlorine is dumped into the water to kill the viruses and bacteria that result from people and the things they leave in public pools (deliberately or not). Would you go over to the edge of the pool with an empty glass, fill it with the pool water and drink it? Of course you wouldn't, so why would you drink tap water with chlorine added?

The picture above shows a simple test you can do to check if there is any chlorine in your tap water. Get three glasses, and put a small amount of tap water in two of them and purified water in the third. In one of the tap water

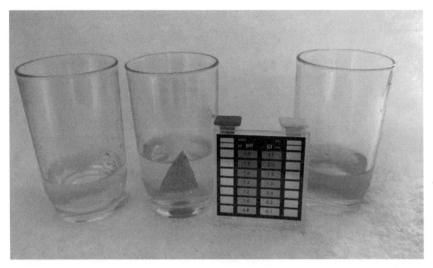

Chlorine test.

glasses place a small segment of apple. In each of the three glasses drop a tablet that tests for chlorine (purchased from Bunnings, your local hardware store or pool supplier) in the water. If there is chlorine in the water it will turn pink. The deeper pink it becomes, the more chlorine is present.

While you can't see it, due to the black and white photo, the glass on the right with only tap water is very pink. The glass on the left with purified water is clear as crystal. What's with the glass in the middle, the one with tap water and food? You will see that the water is almost as clear as the purified water. How can that be? We know there is chlorine in that water, as the glass on the right clearly demonstrates. Why isn't it pink like the other glass? It logically means that there is much less chlorine in the water *and* there is only one other place it could be. Yep, in the apple. In other words, food absorbs chlorine. In other, other words, any food you rinse, soak or cook in tap water will absorb chlorine. In other, other, other words, you and your family will be eating toxic and poisonous foods!

Still not convinced that tap water is toxic and dangerous? Go to your kitchen tap and unscrew the aerator from the end of it and have a look and see what's been trapped in that small space (see the photos below). Yuuuuckk!

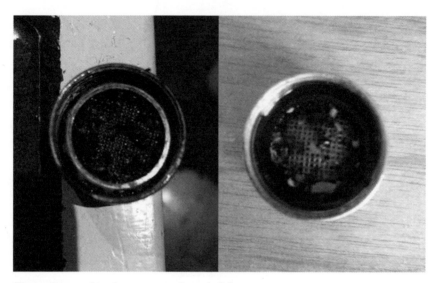

The gunk trapped in the aerator on the end of the tap.

That's just what's been captured; think about what may have actually passed through and collected in the glass that you pour down your throat and into your body.

Do you really still need more reasons to convince yourself to avoid tap water? If you do, let me ask you this: how old is your home? How old are the pipes that funnel the water through the tap and into the glass, pot, kettle or bottle that you eventually put into your fragile body? Do you know what condition those pipes are in? Do you know what the water is collecting as it comes rushing out the end of the tap and into your body?

In the following photo, the section of pipe used to lead to a kitchen tap. Honestly, if you knew your water was passing through a pipe in this condition, would you drink the water or would you allow your children to drink it?

But wait, there's more! My last disgusting photograph was taken when I changed over my water filter. I'm pretty sure you can guess which was the used one. All I can say is, I'm glad that gunk is in the filter and not my body. Make no mistake about it, that muck will be filtered out of the water – either by a quality machine, or by your kidneys and liver. Which would you prefer: to *buy* a filter or *be* a filter?

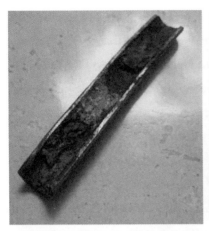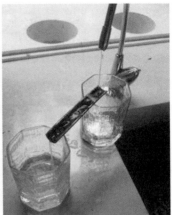

Would you really drink this water?

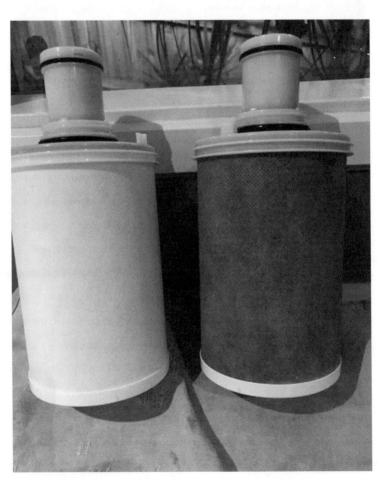

It's better to buy a filter than be a filter!

I hope you can now see that drinking tap water is not an option that will lead to the optimal wellness I'm talking about in this book. It is continual exposure to these chemicals, poisons and toxins that will lead to dis-ease. I urge you to take this seriously and carefully consider the type of water you consume. If you're on the same page as me then you will want to know the alternative options to tap water. If you're not, then you can skip this next bit.

Alternatives to tap water

If you want to find an alternative to tap water, then no doubt you'll consider bottled water. Is it better than tap water? In most cases yes, but as there are no standards for bottled water (in Australia anyway) then often it's really just pot luck. I'm going to try to discourage you from going down the bottled water path for a variety of compelling reasons:

- As I've already mentioned there are no standards for bottled water in Australia, so you really don't know what you're getting. Standards would make manufacturers responsible for producing safe, wholesome and truthfully labelled products.

- The price of bottled water is astronomical. Depending where you purchase, it can potentially be up to ten dollars per litre. Let's be conservative and say you and the family spend just $20 per week on bottled water. That's more than $1,000 per year, every year, forever. That's an amount of money that most families would rather use for something else.

- The leaching of the bottle's plastic into the water you consume and how it will disrupt the body's hormone regulation is something I advise you to research.

- What about our environment? What is happening to the waste products? Where is the plastic being dumped and what is it doing to life on our planet? Again, something I recommend you research.

Got it now: no tap water and no bottled water. So, what does that leave? The best option for your well-being and your back pocket is to get a high-quality water purification system. Yes, I did say back pocket. We discussed that the ongoing and easily measurable cost of bottled water is around one to two thousand dollars per year, depending on how often you purchase. There is no way we can calculate the ongoing cost of drinking polluted and toxic tap water every day, except to say that I guarantee it's a cost that no one wants to pay.

There are many types of water filters and purifiers that range from $20 to $20,000. You don't need to spend $20,000 on a purification system, but don't nickel and dime it either – you will get what you pay for. It's all about understanding the difference between cost and value.

Have you ever been seduced into buying a cheap printer? I have. One day I was standing in the queue at the post office to buy a stamp and I walked out with a name branded printer. I couldn't resist; it was a reputable brand and it was on special at a price that seemed too good to be true. I should've known. The ink was expensive, but it didn't worry me because I was sure it would last all year long – ha ha. Two months later I needed to spend another $150 on ink. Then in two months, guess what? Yes, another $150 and another and another and another! A year later that printer I spent a mere $60 on had cost me almost $2,000 and would continue to cost me that every single year.

I hear you asking: what's this got to do with water purification? That's a great question. People are regularly seduced into buying low-cost water filters, just as I was to buy that printer. The difference is that the cost of buying a cheap filter will be much higher than just the dollar amount. What's at stake is the well-being of you and your family.

Yes, buying the cheap jug filter is better than nothing. Please, however, consider the level and quality of filtration. In other words, what is still left in the water and what's the ongoing cost of replacing filters? Water filters absolutely need to be replaced as directed. The worst thing you can do is continue to drink water through a filter that needs to be replaced and is full of slimy and disgusting gunk. Think about it: if the filter is full and water continues to flow through it, what will happen? Since you've asked, let me tell you: the gunk in the filter will be flushed back out and into the glass, pot or kettle that you will be consuming from. Got the visual?

From a financial perspective, you need to clearly understand the difference between cost and value. The money you invest up front on a quality machine will save you enormously in the future. Laura and I invested in a high-quality unit that purifies the water and lasts for 5,000 litres (1,320 gallons) before the filter needs to be changed – that is 12 to 18 months. We spend only six cents per litre on purified water, and will forever, which is amazing value.

Strategies to increase water consumption

Now we have the type of water you'll drink well and truly sorted, the next discussion is how to drink the amount of water you need to drink for optimal wellness. Remember, this is about feeling, looking and functioning at your very best. This is about living a life with no restrictions and being, doing and having all you want. This is about understanding that your health and well-being is the non-negotiable foundation for ultimate success in life.

Assuming you understand what I'm saying, then now's the time to stop negotiating the price of drinking enough of the right type of water. Now's the time to drink more water. It's really not that hard; it's just a simple decision. Yes, it's hilarious when people joke about the fact that alcohol, coffee and soft drink have lots of water in them. What's not funny is diabetes, liver disease, heart disease and cancer, the inevitable consequences of long-term habitual consumption of these beverages.

Okay, so juice, soft drink, coffee and alcohol may be tastier than water, but as a very wise person once said: 'Sometimes there has to be a purpose greater than taste.' Would you prefer the taste of soft drink or the taste of better well-being? Would you rather the taste of alcohol or the taste of quality time with people you care about? Would you choose the taste of multiple coffees per day or the taste of optimal energy, high productivity and desirable results in life? It's your choice.

Here are some simple and easily implementable strategies to increase water consumption in a busy life, if the choice of optimal well-being is your preference. There is nothing new here, but hopefully you are in a place where you are ready to act on them.

- Focus each morning on why good health and well-being is important to you and look at your vision board.
- Set an actual goal for the amount of pure water you will drink for the day.
- Drink 500 to 1,000 millilitres (17 to 34 fluid ounces) of purified water first thing in the morning before eating any food. Add a squeeze of lemon to add flavour and to alkaline the water. I'll talk more about why this is a particularly great strategy for flushing toxins later in the book.
- Take a glass or stainless steel water bottle with you and keep sipping on it throughout the day.
- Booby-trap yourself for success by planting water bottles in places you frequent: in your home, office, car and so on.
- Set an alarm or some form of notification every hour to remind you to have a drink.
- Eat more foods that have high water content such as salads, vegetables and fruits.
- Every time you drink purified water, imagine a power source entering your body to fuel, hydrate and propel yourself towards greater well-being and a better life.

Water is a magical liquid. Water can give life, protect life and enhance life, so please don't compromise it. Drink enough of the right type of water and experience how it will help you live the life of optimal wellness for which you are striving.

Putting the pieces in place

I was speaking to a group of lawyers at a law firm a few years ago and talking about a range of simple wellness steps that, over time and with daily focus, would create some incredibly positive changes. Among the seven things I outlined that day, one of them was to simply drink an extra 500 millilitres (17 fluid ounces) of purified water each day. I'm sure you'd agree this is something everyone can do.

One lady came to me after the session, thanked me for the talk and then began to justify why six out of the seven things I discussed were not possible for her at that time. She did say, however, she could commit to the extra 500 millilitres of purified water each day. A few weeks later I came back to that same organisation for follow-up purposes and was greeted enthusiastically by this same lady. She looked very different.

Her skin looked clearer, her energy levels were higher and she had even lost some weight. I told her how great she looked and asked her what she had been doing. She went on to explain to me that, while she started with the extra 500 millilitres of purified water per day, she was soon feeling so much better as a result of the increased water intake that she started to implement some of the other strategies. She was eating better and exercising more and had a much more positive attitude than the lady I had met just a few weeks earlier. All this came from a simple decision to drink an extra 500 millilitres of purified water per day.

I think you've got my message from this chapter and I don't want to bore you with more of the same. I hope you will take this on board and start to flood your body each day with two to three litres (67 to 100 fluid ounces) of wonderful life-giving purified water.

 ## Key questions and action steps

1. Do you now understand the importance water plays in your optimal well-being?

2. Start today to add an extra 500 millilitres of pure water into your body each day.

3. If you don't have one and you are convinced that tap water is not the best option, start researching water purification units.

4. If you want more information or any help about finding a high-quality water purification unit, please contact me through the landing page: andrewjobling.com.au/books/wellness-puzzle/.

5

The power of whole food

We hold the cure for modern-day diseases in our hands.
The cure is prevention, not indifference. The cure is pro-action,
not reaction. The cure is real food, not processed food.

Hippocrates of Kos was born in the year 460 BCE. He was a Greek physician and is considered to be one of the most outstanding and influential figures in the history of medicine. I'm not going to go into any detail about his life in this book, except to focus on what is probably his most famous quote: 'Let food be thy medicine and medicine be thy food.'

What a visionary this man was; he knew it over 2,000 years ago. His quote has been known, read and used by a vast majority of the world for all of that time. You and I have heard it many times before, haven't we? When did we stop listening? When did we lose sight of the power, nutrient content, wellness and medicine that comes naturally to us wrapped in the whole foods available for us to consume?

If we would all simply live by this Hippocratean philosophy, and let 'food be thy medicine', I know there would not be the same level of dis-ease we are experiencing in the year 2019 CE and beyond. This chapter is all about inspiring you to return from the dark side – if you've strayed – to the side of light, wellness, purpose and abundance.

Again, I want to emphasise here that I'm not a doctor and I'm not a qualified dietician, nutritionist or naturopath. I am a passionate and concerned observer who has seen, experienced and learned an incredible amount over a 54-year journey on this planet. What I have keenly observed and am most passionate about is what Hippocrates spoke about. He had it spot on 2,500 years ago and is still on the money today: food is a large part of the solution. The only thing Hippocrates may not have foreseen, all those years ago, was that today's food can also be a large part of the problem. I think you know what I'm talking about.

We have all been blessed with an incredible body that has the ability to do so much more than we often believe. It's the vehicle with which we get through life, and it allows us to create the outcomes we desire or it's responsible for a life we don't want. It all depends on how we treat it. The most important thing to realise is that you are the owner and the driver of your body and you are 100 per cent responsible for and in control of where it goes and how it performs.

Your body is the most elaborate and complex piece of equipment on the planet. No machine, computer or device can be manufactured to perform or reproduce even a fraction of what your body is capable of. It can clearly visualise and imagine the life you want. It can create a step-by-step plan for its realisation. It can think, act, move, build, adapt and overcome in order to create an amazing outcome. Your body has the ability to do things so vastly unique that even comprehending them is a mind-blowing concept. Even more amazing news is that you can self-manage, self-heal and self-create your body – that is, if you feed it the raw material it needs.

Imagine a car that self-serviced, dishes that self-cleaned or a bed that self-made? We would all run out and buy them, right? We would love the fact that we could save time and money and have things that just looked after themselves, wouldn't we? Well, you already have it with your body, but I dare say you're taking it for granted. I dare say you're not feeding it what it requires to self-manage. I dare say you're not taking advantage of the most sophisticated and high-level vehicle on the planet. I dare say you are allowing it to run down, get broken and be less than efficient. Do you truly understand that – unlike a car, dish or bed – your body cannot be replaced? Once it's broken, it's broken for good. It's all over, red rover! So, why wouldn't we feed it what it requires?

A car needs quality fuel, oil, fluids and parts to perform at its optimal level. If your income relied on your car being able to get you around, you wouldn't put soda instead of petrol in the fuel tank, beer instead of oil in the engine or sand instead of water in the radiator, would you? A racehorse requires premium feed, the right nutrients, lots of water and adequate rest and recovery. If you wanted to own a champion racehorse, you wouldn't feed it burgers, pizza, ice-cream and beer. That would be crazy, right?

You know where I'm heading with this, don't you? The greatest asset you have is your health. The most prized possession you own is your body. The only way you can ever live the life you dream about is to be optimally healthy. So, what I'm about to say is coming from the right place and meant to help you, even though it may sound harsh. Here it comes: stop treating your body like a garbage dump! Stop filling it with processed food. Stop relying on stimulants rather than good nutrients for energy. Stop putting chemicals, toxins and poisons into the only vehicle you have. Treat your body with the respect it deserves and it will give you everything you desire.

There, I've said my piece! That's enough of that negative stuff; let's talk about some cool, simple and life-changing strategies to help you eat your way back to amazing well-being. Does that sound better?

As you know, I wrote a book in which I outlined a common-sense guide to eating and exercising, which was published back in 2004. Yes, that was a long time ago, but I'm proud that even today, some 15-plus years later,

I still live by the principles I wrote in that book. People's opinions, ideas and philosophies may change – often like the wind – but there are some things that never change. One of those things is that there is no substitute for eating whole foods: fruits, vegetables, whole grains, good fats and quality proteins.

I recently had a meeting with a personal trainer who I'd never met before. As I always do with everyone in the wellness industry I meet, I gave her a copy of my book. Most people I present this gift to are thrilled and grateful: some are indifferent and a few are negative and critical. Guess which one this lady was? Yep, you guessed it. She didn't say 'thank you'; in fact, the first thing she did was to look and see when it was published. She then said, 'It was published in 2004. Do you have anything more recent? This can't be up to date with current research. I don't know what I could do with the book.' To be honest, I was a bit taken aback and stunned for a short time. After I recovered, I asked her a simple question: 'Do you think anything has changed around the concept that eating whole food is the best option?' I tried to speak to her as respectfully as I could when I really wanted to tell her exactly what she could do with the book!

I'm so incredibly passionate about the power of good nutrition, I just wish more people felt the same. Are you? What would it be worth for you to get passionate? What will it cost you if you don't? There is so much time, energy and cost invested in finding cures for modern-day diseases when we hold the cure in our hands. The cure is prevention not indifference. The cure is pro-action, not reaction. The cure is real food, not processed food. Maybe it's time to take our good friend Hippocrates a little more seriously.

Over the next few chapters I'm going to share what I know, what I've learned, what I believe and what I've experienced about good nutrition. Please keep in mind that I'm an ex-footballer, so my way of explaining things is simple and very much in layman's terms. If you want the full scientific description of these concepts then there are other books out there that will do this. My aim is to keep it simple, help you understand, identify potential areas requiring attention and inspire you to do something positive.

There are problems, issues and challenges affecting our eating habits in the 21st century that seem to be recurring and leading many people down a very predictable and unsavoury path. It is my belief that, if you understand what's happening, why it's happening and how to fix it, then you can take control of your wellness and not have to rely on anyone or anything else. How does that sound? You hold the key to your wellness in your hands, and all it takes is the right knowledge and attitude and positive action.

To work out how to improve things, we need to look at when they started going bad. Coincidentally (or not), this happened as soon as we started tampering with our food sources. Let's face it, our ancestors had many issues to contend with, but heart disease, cancers, type II diabetes, depression, anxiety, inflammation and many other of the rampant modern concerns were not in the mix. When life was simpler people's purpose was clearer, and eating real food, drinking pure water, breathing clean air and the same modern-day challenges were non- or rarely existent.

This next section is again taken from my book on sensible eating and exercising.

In a Perfect World

Paul Chek in his book/CD pack, *You Are What You Eat*, describes the 'Wheel of Life'. Simply put, it explains the cycle of life and nutrients from plant to animal to humankind to soil and back to plant.

In a perfect world, plants grow in soil that is nutrient-rich and devoid of any pollutants. The pests are controlled through natural means such as ladybugs and birds, and fertilisation occurs naturally through the decomposition of natural matter with the help of earthworms. The plants and soil receive water that is free from pollutants, even further enhancing the health of the plant.

Animals feed from the healthy, nutrient-rich plants and drink the pure and plentiful water. They grow naturally and with optimal health; their only major concern being their predators, of which humans are one.

The humans eat the natural, nutrient-rich plants and the flesh of the healthy animals. Their bodies grow strong, function well and are able to fight off any infection or other disorder with ease before it can become a long-term problem. Full of energy, the humans are more motivated, more productive and they lead longer, more fulfilling and happier lives. Eventually they invent the TV with remote control and couldn't be happier!!

As the plant and animal life die they decompose to further enrich the soil. They create an environment for the earthworms to survive, thrive, turn and aerate the soil. The worms help to create compost, which is ideal food for the microorganisms in the soil, which provide the nutrient-rich food for the plants. And the cycle repeats.

How Did Things Ever Get So Bad?

The population expanded, technology exploded, the demand for food and consumables grew, the need to produce more food at a faster rate created a need for processing, preserving and modifying foods. Chemicals were added to plants to make them grow faster, bigger and stronger. Chemicals were added to the soil and plants to kill and deter pests, or to fertilize the soil.

Unfortunately, what was not considered was that all these chemicals were and still are killing all the vital micro-organisms and essential nutrients in the soil. Leaving nothing but a barren and lifeless soil full of harmful chemicals to be passed on to any plant grown in it, and consequently to any animal eating it.

Now consider the modern day 'Wheel of Life'. Plants grow in soil that is nutrient deficient thus producing plants that are nutrient deficient. Chemicals, insecticides, fungicides, fertilizers added to plants and soil further create very undesirable produce. The crops are nourished with water that contains a variety of environmental pollutants, chemicals and bacteria.

The farmed animals are fed these grains and plants and consequently become nutrient deficient and affected from taking in a variety of chemicals. This affects the growth and health of the animals. They get sick and so are treated with antibiotics and other synthetic medications, which not only kill infection, but also affect the quality of the muscle (which we will eat). Many animals are kept under inhumane conditions and fed synthetic supplements to enhance growth to cater to the growing demands of the marketplace.

We humans now consume these plants and animals that are in such a bad state and as a result, we lack energy, have trouble staying in shape, we are more prone to disease, we spend more time and money on the doctors and the quality of our life is seriously affected. The worst news is that we are less motivated, less productive, achieve less and therefore take a lot longer before we can afford the big screen TV with the remote control!

My goal is to help you regain the benefits from the positive cycle of life, so let's make a deal. I will give you the basic knowledge, ideas and strategies to create this positive cycle. You will need to be honest with yourself, learn them, apply them and create positive habits. Is it a deal? Okay; let's do this thing!

Over the next six chapters I'm going to discuss my observations of, understanding of and experiences about what I believe to be the key areas of 21st century nutritional concerns, all of which have been significantly impacted through the industrial age and processing of foods. Anyone over 40 years of age has seen this negative cycle evolve.

We wanted to lose weight, so we processed food to remove the fat and added sugar as an alternative and ended up getting fatter. Then we realised that too much sugar was no good, so we processed that food even more to remove the sugar. We replaced it with synthetically produced sweetener and we got sicker. We wanted more convenience, had higher demands and required food to last longer on the supermarket shelves. Consequently, we created trans fats, artificial colours, flavours and preservatives and we got more lethargic, more allergic, more stressed, fatter and sicker.

The crazy thing is that we know more now about good nutrition than we ever have. We have easy access to all the information we need at any time of the night and day. Yet, day by day, week by week, month by month and year by year we are getting sicker and more devastated by poor health. Now is the time for you – yes, YOU – to take control. Not just for your sake, but for the sake of your children and the generations to come. The decisions you make and actions you take today will change generations, so make the best decisions you can make and take the actions you know you should be taking.

Here are three simple steps I'm going to expand on over the next few chapters. *Step one* is to get back to eating whole food. That's real food, not processed, packaged or tampered with food. *Step two* is to enjoy the taste of great food, good nutrition and optimal well-being. *Step three* is to supplement in any areas that require a higher level of nutrition. I will expand and unpack these as we go on our gastronomic journey together.

The basics are known by us all. In general terms, you know what you should be doing and how you should be eating, right? There are subtle things, however, that may not be obvious that I want to make sure you fully understand. Things such as how to create and maintain a metabolism that works for you, not against you. Things such as the importance of your cellular health and how to have healthy cells and a healthy body. Things such as the impact stress is having on your well-being and some cool nutritional solutions. Things such as gut health and how to keep the good stuff in and get the bad stuff out. Through understanding and awareness comes empowerment.

Are you ready for some fun? Are you ready to understand how to get your health back and/or take it to the next level? Are you ready to look and feel fantastic? Are you ready to feel excited and empowered to take control of your well-being?

Great, then let's get going!

Putting the pieces in place

As a first step in the process of hitting 'refresh' of your eating to truly allow food to *be thy medicine*, I want to encourage you to eat food in or as close as possible to its natural state. Corn on the cob would be a better option than Cornflakes, Froot Loops are not real fruit and Nutri-Grain is definitely not iron man food. Eat real fruits, vegetables, whole grains and quality protein. You know that already, don't you?

Let's go back to Sherry Strong's nature principle, which she explains in a really cool and understandable way. Her principle states that the easier it is to obtain a food in nature the healthier, more nutritious and life giving it will be for you. For example, if you are trying to decide the healthiest and best option between fresh or canned pineapple, then just think about which would be easier to obtain. Now, I know the jokers reading this will say it's easier to just go to the supermarket and buy a can of pineapple. Ha ha ha! But let's say you were on a desert island, which then would be easier to obtain? Would it be easier to climb the tree to get the pineapple, peel it, slice it, mix up sugar syrup, make the can from scratch, place the pineapple pieces and syrup into the can, seal the can then open it again and eat it, OR just climb the tree, get the pineapple, peel it, slice it and eat it? Obvious answer!

What about the chicken or the egg: which would be healthier? The answer can be discovered simply through a logical thought process. Which would be easier to obtain if you were in nature? You could locate a chicken, try to catch it then kill it, pluck it, gut it, chop it, cook it and eat it, OR you could simply find the chicken's nest and take the egg. Do you understand the principle?

Eat whole food and the benefits you will immediately start to notice will transform the way you look and feel and the life you can live. Start letting food be thy medicine and medicine be thy food!

 ## Key questions and action steps

1. Would it be worth it for you to start making some changes in the way you are eating?

2. What simple substitutions could you make to move from processed foods back to more natural and whole foods?

3. What are your favourite fruits and vegetables? Eat more of them.

4. Do you truly know the source of the food you are eating and the process it's been through by the time it gets onto your plate?

5. Are you aware of the impact processed food is having on your health and the health of your family?

6. Read carefully the next few chapters and please make the changes that you need to make to live the life you desire.

The power of whole food
Get the metabolic fire burning

The only answer, if being optimally lean, fit and healthy for life is your goal, is to develop a sound, healthy and enjoyable eating regime that creates a strong metabolic fire, one you can maintain.

Have you ever been camping? I think we all have at some stage in our life. Some people love it and get out in the great outdoors regularly. My idea of camping is four stars! One of the key activities when camping is to build, light and maintain a healthy campfire. It's needed for warmth, for light at night and to cook food, so it's a pretty important part of the camping experience.

My understanding is that it's simple really; you just get some wood, light it and it burns all day and all night long. Right? Of course not, and I'm sure the avid campers and fire starters reading this will correct me if I'm wrong, but a good campfire requires quality fuel, time, energy and attention. Hmmm, sounds familiar to me …

You need solid dry wood, twigs and some leaves or paper. You need to get it started with the leaves or paper and then add the twigs. As it starts burning, you need to add some more substantial wood. If you want to keep it burning strong, you need to add fuel to it regularly, probably every 30 to 60 minutes. What's lighting and maintaining a campfire got to do with good nutrition? The answer is: everything!

We have all heard about metabolism and its importance, but do you really understand it and are you looking after yours? Again, I'm going to put this as simply as I can: metabolism is the rate at which your body does stuff; 'stuff' being the scientific term. The rate at which your body burns fat is determined by metabolism. The rate at which your body produces energy is controlled largely by metabolism. The rate at which your body can heal itself is regulated by metabolism. So the first step in restoring and optimising your well-being through nutrition is to get your metabolism burning strong.

There are several things that will impact your metabolism but I'll just refer to three. The first is your age. As you age, your metabolism will naturally slow. Are you getting younger? If you follow the principles in this book you'll hopefully feel younger and live longer, but like me you are getting older each day. Hence, we can't control this one so let's put it aside for now.

The second thing that impacts metabolism is exercise. It is believed by many, even me for a period of time, that exercise will improve metabolic rate. Is that your understanding? Well, that's an interesting one that I'd like to explore with you right now. The short answer is that exercise *will* improve metabolism, on the condition that you have a solid nutritional foundation.

Here's the long answer to help you understand this. Have you ever heard that to lose weight you simply need to eat less and exercise more? Have you ever been told that it's a straightforward equation: less calories going in and more caloric expenditure equates to weight loss? Heard it? Believe it? Open and willing to question it? Have you tried it? How did it work for you, long term, I mean? If you're like most people who follow this diet mentality and approach, you probably lost weight and then put it all back on, plus more, at some later stage. Am I right? Would you like to know why?

As I explain this, I would like to introduce the third and most important thing that impacts metabolism, which is nutrition. The body has three main fuel sources it can tap into: carbohydrates, fat and protein. Its preferred source is carbohydrates. In a dieting situation or when you skip meals, either deliberately or not, you simply reduce the amount of food and often the carbohydrates you consume, right? In conjunction with this, if you are trying to lose weight, you may increase your exercise and energy expenditure. Done it before? As a result, the body goes into an energy deficit. In other words, it's expending more energy than it is receiving and, therefore, needs to find energy from elsewhere.

If there's not enough energy coming from carbohydrates, the body starts tapping into its second option: fat stores. That sounds good, doesn't it? Well, it is good for about three days and no more. Your body is very clever; it wants to keep you alive and it doesn't care how you look or feel. After three days of restricted calories and/or too much exercise the body goes into starvation mode, which is obviously not good. Its sole purpose now is survival, so it will stop burning fat and start storing it for long-term survival. It will then start breaking down muscle, converting it to protein and using that for energy.

Losing muscle may seem like a good thing because the scales will be heading in the right direction, but it's actually the worst thing you can do for your body if having energy and being lean and healthy is the goal. When you lose muscle, your metabolism will slow down because a large part of your metabolic rate is determined by lean muscle. It is inside the muscle cell where you burn fat. Less muscle means you will burn less fat, and when you go off the diet – and you will, because the alternative is death by malnutrition – you will put all the weight back on plus more and it will be much harder to get rid of.

I met a lady not long ago, at a talk I was giving on this very topic, who told me she'd lost 16 kilograms (35 pounds) on a popular weight-loss program. It was a calorie-restricted and largely starvation diet. After I complimented her on her impressive achievement, she replied, 'It would have been more impressive if I didn't put 23 kilograms [51 pounds] back on.'

She lost muscle so her metabolism slowed down, and when she went off the diet and started eating more food her body had no option but to store it as fat. Please hear this and hear this well: diets don't work and will never work if being optimally lean, fit and healthy for life is your goal. The only answer is to develop a sound, healthy and enjoyable eating regime that creates a strong metabolic fire, one you can maintain. That's what I'm about to share with you.

Let's run with the campfire metaphor, as it's one we can all understand. If you were camping out in wild terrain in inclement conditions and you woke up at the break of dawn and were cold and hungry, how long would you wait to start the fire? Five minutes, 10 minutes, 30 minutes, an hour, two hours or more? I'm guessing you would get it started as soon as possible, within 10 to 15 minutes, to get you warm. Would I be right?

Please don't be offended if I'm talking about you right now. Do, however, take notice. It's crazy that so many people get up and then wait up to two or three hours before eating. If this is you, please understand the devastating impact waiting so long to put fuel in your body is having on your life – yes, your life. By skipping the most important meal of the day your metabolism stays low, your energy levels are compromised, your moods are affected, your decision making is impacted and your concentration is diminished. You will crave and make poor food choices, rely on stimulants, eat too much at the wrong end of the day, gain weight, lack nutrients, have a higher risk of chronic disease and your life will be less than it could be. All this from skipping breakfast? My answer is a resounding YES!

If the *only* decision you make after reading this entire book is to eat something within 10 to 15 minutes of getting out of bed, your metabolic fire will be started and most of the things I have listed above will be prevented. That one simple decision will help you to have more energy, lose more fat and be healthier and happier. Would it be worth it?

Many people love to argue with me and are convinced they eat breakfast. So let's clear this up right now: if you get up at 6 am and eat at 9 am, 8 am or even 7 am, that's not breakfast. You have officially missed the most important meal, and will set off a potentially devastating domino effect to impact your day and your life. *Eat something natural and healthy within fifteen minutes of getting out of bed.*

If I were starting a campfire I would use twigs and newspaper to get a flame burning. I suggest burning the newspaper before you actually read it! Then within a few of minutes I would put some slightly larger pieces of wood on it to keep it burning longer and stronger. Agree? That's exactly what I suggest you do as soon as you get up. No, I don't mean eat paper and twigs; I do mean eat something light, natural and with a high glycaemic index to get your blood sugars up and your fire started.

My suggestion is to eat a small amount of fruit such as watermelon or pineapple, then within five to 10 minutes eat something more substantial with protein included. This could be a slice of wholegrain bread with a poached egg on top, some natural muesli with protein powder and natural yoghurt, or it could be a yummy smoothie with fruit, protein powder, nuts, seeds and yoghurt. The protein is important as it slows the release of sugar into the system, regulates blood sugar levels and keeps you feeling sustained. This is just as a larger piece of wood on the fire will keep it burning for longer.

Once your fire is burning, should you just assume it will keep burning? Of course not, just as you should never assume, because you've had a good breakfast, you don't need to eat anything until dinner. The only way to keep a fire burning strong and hot is to put quality fuel on it every hour or so. My recommendation is that you go with the same concept as an eating strategy: put some quality fuel into your body every 60 to 90 minutes. Yes, you heard me right; every 60 to 90 minutes!

You may be thinking you couldn't possibly eat that much food. If you are, let's clear this one up right now. Think about your current eating habits. The first question I have for you is, are they giving you the results you want with your health, energy and body? If not, would you be open to try something different? If so, then let me ask you this: when do you eat most of the food in your day? Is it in the afternoon and evening? Do you ever over-eat or make poor choices because you are starving and/or craving?

No matter what results you're getting with your food, it's because you have created your own regime or habit of eating. Unfortunately, most people unconsciously develop very negative and destructive habits that take them down an undesirable path. Many people I speak to skip breakfast for a multitude of reasons: they get up too late and are rushing, they are not hungry at that time of the day, they erroneously believe skipping breakfast is a good way to lose weight and they often, and unknowingly, start their day significantly behind the eight ball.

This is what generally happens: people rush out the door with no food but a cup of coffee. Coffee, while a stimulant, will have a detrimental impact on blood sugar, hence energy levels during the day. People get themselves through the morning on caffeine, and perhaps high-sugar snacks such as biscuits, bars or bread. This throws the blood sugar levels into a chaotic roller coaster, sending it up and then down, leading to fatigue, low moods, poor concentration and cravings.

As you can imagine or may have experienced, when you're craving it is very difficult to make good choices. The day is often littered with processed foods, sugary snacks and coffee to try to keep going. Later in the afternoon and evening, with low blood sugar levels and lower resistance, over-eating – even bingeing – can be the result. Eating a large dinner, dessert and then going to bed with a very full stomach leaves the body processing and digesting food all night, which uses a lot of the body's energy stores and causes weight gain. In the morning it's not unusual to wake up tired and with no appetite, and the whole negative pattern repeats itself. Do you relate to this at all?

This pattern can be changed very simply and powerfully, and when it is it will make all the difference in the world. Eating breakfast then eating small meals throughout the day will keep the fire and energy burning. You will feel better, be more energised, have more focus, be in better moods, make more desirable food choices, eat less in the evening, sleep more soundly and wake up energised, hungry and ready to go again. Doesn't that sound like a better option?

If you were to take all the food you are currently consuming and distribute it evenly – eating small portions every 60 to 90 minutes – throughout the day rather than in two or three large meals, could you see how this might work? Your body is more readily able to handle smaller quantities more regularly consumed than it is to eating larger meals less frequently. By adding a small amount of protein and some highly nutritious fruits, vegetables, good fats and whole grains with each meal and snack, you will turn your body into a metabolically charged fat-burning, energy-producing and immunity-building machine.

To help you visualise what I'm talking about here, I will give you a sample of a typical day of eating for me so you understand that eating every 60 to 90 minutes is not that big a deal. I will also say that eating regularly is not hard for me any more because my body now tells me, like an alarm, when it's time for fuel. Your body, as mine, will remind you like clockwork when you have created the right habits.

Time	Meal	Comments
0600	Small piece of pineapple	*Starts the fire and gets it flaming.*
0610	A few segments of mandarin and a couple of raw nuts or half a protein bar	*Keeps it burning, but is not too heavy on my stomach for exercise.*
0615	Exercise session	
0700	Small piece of pineapple	*Gets the fire flaming again.*

Time	Meal	Comments
0710	Small bowl of natural muesli with protein powder, berries and coconut milk	*The combination of whole grains, fruit and protein makes it a sustainable and satisfying fuel source.*
0830	Quality protein bar	*Tastes good and is convenient, and quality ones will provide the right ratio of protein and good fats and will be low in carbohydrates. They keep the fire burning.*
0945	A couple of carrot and celery sticks and a boiled egg	*Provides nutrients and is a good combination of carbohydrates and protein.*
1100	A small handful of raw nuts	*They have protein, good fats and quality carbohydrates. My favourites are almonds, brazil nuts, walnuts and macadamias.*
1230	Three-egg omelette with diced tomato, Brussels sprouts, cauliflower and mushrooms, followed by half a mandarin	*Yummy! I don't have bread with this; I don't need it.*
1400	Protein shake with nuts, berries and natural yoghurt	*Simple, nutritious and delicious.*
1515	A few raw nuts	*Fire still burning strong.*
1630	Half a protein bar	*As above.*
1800	Vegetables steamed or stir fried with chicken, meat or fish or a salad with chicken, meat or fish, followed by the other half of the mandarin	*This is a light meal and I rarely have bread, rice or pasta. As I eat regularly all day I don't need a large meal.*

Time	Meal	Comments
1930	Half a protein bar	*The other half.*
2045	A little bit of dark chocolate	*Mmmmm!*
2 x day	Supplements: vitamins, minerals and omega-3	*I'll discuss this in later chapters.*
Drink	Throughout the day: herbal tea occasionally and two to three litres (67 to 100 fluid ounces) of purified water	*I've never had a cup of coffee in my life, so I can't see a reason to start now. I don't need another addiction!*

Keep in mind this is just an example of my day. If you think I'm suggesting I never eat pizza, pasta, chocolate, ice-cream or any other yummy indulgence, you're wrong. If you think I'm a saint and never drink alcohol, again you're wrong. Like everyone, I love my occasional indulgence. The key to me being lean and healthy at 54 is creating good habits, so when I treat myself to yummy indulgences it's because I want and enjoy them, not because I'm craving them. In this way, it's easy to not have to try and rely on the myth of w-i-l-l-p-o-w-e-r, but instead practise that scary word m-o-d-e-r-a-t-i-o-n. It's easy if you get your metabolic fire burning.

As you may know, hunger, cravings and over-eating are primary issues these days for many people. What you may not know is that they can be solved easily by eating the right sorts of foods regularly. Sometimes, however, working out what is the right food can be more challenging, due to very clever media and marketing. The main reason over-eating is such a large problem is because of the lack of nutrient value in much of the food we eat, so our bodies craves more.

One of the indulgences I enjoy is yum cha. I don't have it often, but when I do I scoff down lots of yummy dumplings in a short period of time. Within about 15 minutes I'm always full to the brim, ready to explode, can hardly move and feel like I won't be able to eat again for weeks. Why is it that within the next hour I'm hungry again? Simple: there are ZERO nutrients in those yum cha dumplings. My body is saying, 'Great, you've just filled me up with nutrient-devoid food. When can I have something that will fuel me, heal me and help me?' My body wants nutrients, not siu mai.

When we eat any processed, fast or nutrient-deficient foods frequently we are prone to over-eating. Why? Because our body will keep craving more until it gets the nutrients it needs. The simple solution is to eat small nutrient-rich meals or snacks on a regular basis and you will solve the craving and over-eating issue by giving your body what it needs. Then you can enjoy your yum cha or other indulgence in moderation.

Start that metabolic fire and keep it burning strong all day, and you won't believe the difference it will make to your health, energy, body fat and every aspect of your life.

Putting the pieces in place

What I'm talking about in this chapter is developing a healthy structure, pattern or habit of eating. As you may have heard me mention once or twice, the wellness outcome you will get is the end product of small, seemingly insignificant actions you take on a daily and weekly basis – those that become unconscious habits. It is simple habits that are the secret to your success but may also be the reason for your decline, so choose your actions wisely.

Once the rhythm of eating breakfast and then regularly throughout the day is created, all that's left is to make sure the food you eat will, as Hippocrates put it so eloquently, be thy medicine. Look for and consume primarily nutrient-rich foods, plant-based carbohydrates, natural grains, quality proteins and good fats. This is nothing new, is it? What I hope is that over the next couple of chapters, as we unpack this nutritional piece to the wellness puzzle in more detail, you will take what is now knowledge and pro-actively and passionately implement it into your daily life.

Key questions and action steps

1. Based on what you now know, how would you rate your metabolic fire?

2. What do you need to do to get it burning strong and working for you?

3. Would you be willing to eat something within 10 to 15 minutes of getting out of bed for one week?

4. Can you see how small regular snacks will be beneficial for you?

5. How important is your dream, your career, your energy and your family? Is it worth making some changes? I hope so.

5

The power of whole food
Cellular health: protect your unit of life

Your cells are your units of life. They are powerful yet sensitive,
they are responsive yet vulnerable. They are your responsibility
to care for, so please do so.

An electronic circuit board is made up of many single components. A building is made up of many single bricks. A community is made up of many single people. The human body is made up of many single cells, in fact, around 37 trillion single cells.

We know what will happen to an electronic circuit board if we remove or damage just one of the components: the circuit board will not function. If any of the bricks in a building are weak, cracked or missing, then the structural integrity of the entire building will be compromised and, over time, may be reduced to rubble. Just one bad, toxic or negative person in a community who influences others could start a domino effect that impacts the entire community and puts it at risk of crumbling.

These are just a few simple analogies to help me emphasise the importance of the health of each single cell in your body. You are cells, that's it! Skin cells, blood cells, muscle cells, fat cells and any other type of cells you can think of. Thirty-seven trillion of them make up your entire body. That being the case, you may be thinking: what would it matter if a few got damaged? That's a good question, and I have an even better answer.

The cells in a human body replicate and replace themselves many times over during the course of a life. Literally speaking, you are not the same person you were last year, because all of the cells that made up your body regenerated and replicated and, over time, were replaced. No matter the state of your cells, they replicate. In other words, a healthy cell replicates to form a healthy cell and an unhealthy cell replicates to form an unhealthy cell.

Okay, let's consider this scenario: for whatever reason, you happen to have one damaged cell. If that cell replicates itself, how many damaged cells do you now have? Correct, you now have two. If those two cells replicate, how many do you have? Yes, the answer is four. Now imagine if this process repeated every day for 31 days. Do you have any idea how many damaged cells you would end up with? If you simply continue to double the previous number 31 times, the answer you will get is well over 10 million! Yes, that would mean 10 million damaged cells. Do you think that may have some impact on your health?

Can you see the importance of every single unit? Every component is critical for an effectively functioning circuit board. Every single brick is needed to be solid to ensure a strong and stable building. Every single person is important in the fabric that makes up every happy and healthy community around the world. Every single cell is essential to keep you strong, happy and healthy.

I'm now about to get as scientific as I am able to or actually want to. The human cell is an incredibly sophisticated and complex structure, yet its role is quite simple.

The three key components of the cell I will discuss are the nucleus, the mitochondria and the cell membrane. Are you ready for my layman

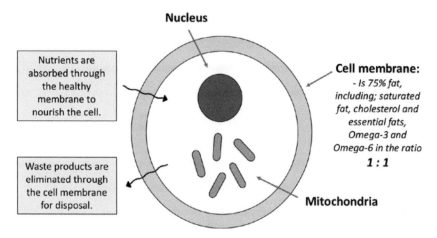

Energised and healthy cell.

definitions of these? Again, if you want to get more into the science and detailed understanding of the human cells this is not the book for you. I want you to have a basic and practical understanding of how they impact YOU and your health, not a scientific understanding. I hope that's okay with you.

The **nucleus** is the brain of the cell. It contains your DNA, which determines your physical character traits, your genetic blueprint and your predisposition to certain conditions. The **mitochondria** is the engine room of the cell. It's where all the chemical reactions take place, the energy is produced, the fat is metabolised and the immune system is fortified. The **cell membrane** is the wall of the cell. It's made of a semi-permeable substance that keeps the cell protected, but also allows for the passage of nutrients in to nourish it and the removal of waste products.

As you can see all three have critical roles in ensuring a healthy body. I want to ask you a question and get you thinking a little. Which of the three do you think is most vulnerable and will have the greatest impact on your optimal well-being?

Is it the nucleus? Let's face it, it holds your DNA and is the brain of your cell and hence your body. Is it the mitochondria? There's a good argument for this: it determines energy levels and fat-burning ability and largely impacts the immune system. Or is it the cell membrane? This is the doorway for nutrients to enter the body to impact the mitochondria and the nucleus, and is the pathway for waste products to exit.

In my opinion, it's the cell membrane that is most vulnerable, because it's hugely influenced by what we consume and is the one component that will have the greatest impact on what happens inside the cell. To me, it's the part of the cell you can and need to look after the most. The chances are that, without even realising what you're doing, you are compromising your cell membranes, hence the health of your cells and therefore your own well-being.

Let's do a quick check. Are you ever tired and lethargic? Do you have trouble moving stubborn fat? Are you prone to sickness at different times? Do you suffer from any inflammation: swelling, skin issues, respiratory conditions, heart issues or anything else similar? Do you have cholesterol or blood pressure issues? If you answered yes to one or more of those questions, the chances are it's because, without even knowing it, you are damaging your cell membranes and reducing their ability to do their job. This may well be because of what you are eating.

The health (composition) of your cell membranes determines their ability to allow nutrients in and move waste products out. It is this that basically controls the function, effectiveness and health of the cells. The great news is that the composition of your cell membranes is controlled by what you eat. In other words, the health of your cells is up to you. Isn't that exciting and empowering? Now, you just need to know how.

As you can see from the diagram, the cell membrane is comprised of around 75 per cent fat. Fat is a strong enough substance to protect the cells and is permeable enough to facilitate the inward passage of nutrients and the removal of waste products. The biggest challenge for your cell membranes is their vulnerability to exposure to the fats you consume. There are several different types of fat, some incredibly beneficial and others devastatingly detrimental.

A healthy and fully functioning cell membrane is composed of a healthy range and balance of fats, including saturated fat, cholesterol, omega-3 and omega-6 fats. Yes, I did say saturated fats and cholesterol. We've been told for so long now to avoid saturated fats and cholesterol and, for about that same period of time, our health in general has declined. Hmmm, I wonder if there's something in that?

It's actually okay for you to eat some animal fat in moderation. It's okay to consume full cream milk, yoghurt and dairy if you like those and have no allergies or intolerances. It's okay to eat butter but *not* margarine. It's okay to eat eggs, and the yolk. In fact, it's much better for you and your cell membranes to eat these types of fats rather than processed versions.

I can remember when I again started eating chicken fat, the tail on my lamb chop and even some pork crackling. It was like coming home! I'm not talking about every day and I'm not talking about overdoing it, so please don't go around telling everyone that Andrew has given you permission to gorge on saturated fat. However, some animal fat in moderation tastes amazing and is necessary for a healthy cell membrane.

Did you know that the difference in fat content between low fat/skim dairy and full cream is almost negligible? The question I would like answered is: what has been done to remove or reduce the natural fat from these products and what impact is it having on our taste buds, our health and the health of our cell membranes? If you do eat and enjoy dairy products in moderation, I want to encourage you to go back to full cream milk, yoghurt, cheese and, dare I say it, ice-cream. Please eat butter, not margarine which is a trans-fat; I'll explain why later in the chapter. Again, this is not an open slather opportunity for you to eat ice-cream every day and overdo dairy products. Please understand my point: the more natural and less processed is the food you consume, the better it will be for you and your cells.

What about eggs? Eggs are such an amazing source of protein, a very healthy source of good cholesterol, are nutrient rich yet are one of the most misunderstood and condemned foods on the planet. We get told to not eat too many eggs. We are instructed to take the yolk out and eat only the egg whites. We get convinced they increase cholesterol, which leads to heart disease. Consequently, we are missing out on some of the greatest taste and wellness benefits available.

Eggs are actually one of nature's incredible superfoods and a critical part of a healthy cell membrane. In an eggshell, eggs increase the portion of healthy protective cholesterol and, at the same time, decrease the unhealthy cholesterol in the body. Eggs are one of the most nutrient-dense foods available. One egg provides 13 essential nutrients (all in the yolk). Eggs are a great source of vitamins A, C, D and E. Eggs are rich in iodine and are a terrific source of anti-oxidants. There is no reason to limit eggs to two to three per week. In fact, two to three per day will have far greater benefit to your health.*

I don't work for the egg board and I'm not getting paid endorsements; I just love eggs! In fact, I had a beautiful three-egg omelette today for lunch with diced Brussels sprouts, cauliflower and tomato. Delicious and nutritious, but enough about eggs.

The fats that have the greatest impact on the effectiveness of the cell membrane are the essential fatty acids: omega-3 and omega-6. They are called essential fats because they cannot be made by the body; they must be consumed. Can you now see how your eating plays such an important role in the health of your cell membranes?

These essential fats must be consumed in a healthy balance and very similar ratio (as you can see illustrated in the earlier diagram). Why? Because they have opposing roles and any imbalance will cause problems, as it is currently doing in the lives of many people. In fact, it's one of the biggest barriers to wellness on the planet at this present time. Let's explore why and how to fix it.

Omega-6 causes inflammation in the body and omega-3 reduces it. Omega-6 is sourced from vegetable oils, which is included in many foods we currently over-consume: fruits, vegetables, grains, carbohydrates, bread, pasta, rice, nuts and seeds. Omega-3 is much harder to source and consequently we

---

*Sourced from https://chriskresser.com/three-eggs-a-day-keep-the-doctor-away/.

eat much less of it. It is sourced in foods such as deep sea cold water fatty fish, flaxseed oil, many leafy greens and a limited number of nuts. Can you see a potential imbalance in your omega-3 to omega-6 ratio, which ideally should be one to one?

Imagine a set of scales. On one side of the scales place all the omega-6–containing fatty foods you eat in one week, and on the other place all the omega-3–containing fatty foods you consume. In other words, compare your weekly consumption of fruits, vegetables, grains, carbohydrates, bread, pasta, rice, nuts and seeds with that of deep sea cold water fatty fish, flaxseed oil and leafy greens. What would your scales be doing? Would they be weighing heavily on the side of omega-6? What do you think your omega-6 to omega-3 ratio really is? Because it certainly isn't one to one, is it? Is it five to one, 10 to one, 20 to one or more? In many cases for most people the ratio is way more than 20 to one in favour of omega-6 fats. This is a serious issue that requires immediate attention.

If you are consuming an abundant imbalance of inflammatory omega-6 fats, what do you think the impact on your body will be? Your body will be in a state of inflammation, resulting in the potential for multiple inflammatory issues such as swelling, high blood pressure, heart issues, eczema, psoriasis, asthma, arthritis, obesity, lethargy, insulin resistance and even type II diabetes. Do any of these conditions affect or concern you? Let me explain what is happening to cause these things.

But before I do, I need to discuss one other type of fat that is having a devastating effect on cell membranes and the health of many people. Back in the mid 1900s as the population started to explode, the mouths we needed to feed began to increase and the demand for food sources to be produced and preserved was becoming more critical. At that time, a fat was created. This fat was synthetically produced to be cheaper to use on a large scale, to enhance taste and to increase the shelf life of the food.

It's called trans fat, and it is used in almost all processed, packaged, bakery and convenience foods. The idea behind it was a noble one. What no one realised at the time, however, was the devastating impact trans fat would have on our health. World-renowned cardiologist Dr Ross Walker, in his book *The Cell Factor*, states that a two per cent increase in consumption of trans fat will increase the risk of heart disease and diabetes by 93 per cent. In this period of history, and as you are reading this book, understand you have a choice. Food can be thy medicine or food can be thy poison; it's up to you to gain the knowledge that will inform your life and enable you to make the choices you need to make.

Trans fat is created when healthy fats are taken through a chemical process called hydrogenation. It synthetically transforms a fat, that is, a liquid at room temperature, and turns it into a solid, totally changing the chemical structure. Margarine is a trans fat, because it starts as a healthy oil and is converted into a solid through this chemical process.

Trans fat has the effect of hardening foods. When you are eating potato chips, biscuits, crackers, cookies and bakery products, what is it mostly about those foods, apart from taste, you enjoy? Is it the crispiness, the crunch and the crackle? Unfortunately, it's that same property of the food that is taking you down a very dangerous path.

Why? Because just as eating too much inflammation-producing omega-6 fats will cause inflammation in the body, so too does eating even a small amount of trans fat cause hardening. Hardening of what? I hear you ask. Let's get back to the vital cell and its membrane and find out.

To quickly recap, a healthy cell membrane needs to be strong, soft, permeable and pliable to allow the passage of nutrients into the cell to nourish it and waste products to be effectively eliminated. A healthy cell membrane is seventy-five per cent fat, including some saturated fat, cholesterol and an equal balance of omega-3 and omega-6 fats. The composition and health of your cell membrane will be determined by the fats you consume. So, the question you need to ask yourself now is: what fats am I consuming and what impact are they having on my cells?

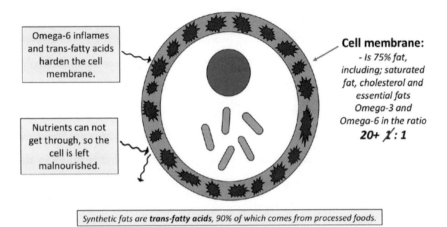

Omega-6 inflames and trans-fatty acids harden the cell membrane.

Cell membrane:
- Is 75% fat, including; saturated fat, cholesterol and essential fats Omega-3 and Omega-6 in the ratio
20+ 1 : 1

Nutrients can not get through, so the cell is left malnourished.

*Synthetic fats are **trans-fatty acids**, 90% of which comes from processed foods.*

Compromised and unhealthy cell.

In the modern day many people over-consume omega-6 fats and processed foods, would you agree? Therefore, it is primarily these two types of fat that enter the body and impact the cell membranes: omega-6, which causes inflammation, and trans fat, which causes hardening. This being the case, what's happening to the cell membranes of the person with these eating habits? Let's explore this.

Over-consumption of omega-6 fats causes the membranes to become inflamed. Over-consumption of processed foods with trans fat causes hardening of the membranes. Can you see how this will devastate the cells' ability to function? The inflamed and hardened membranes inhibit the passage of nutrients to enter and nourish the cell.

The result of this is malnourished cells, which will lead to lethargy, low immunity and cravings. Have you ever craved before? Do you crave Brussels sprouts? I think not. You crave sugar, right? This craving and desperate need to get energy leads many people to make choices they know, deep down, are wrong choices, but they make them anyway. Why? Cravings lead to an emotional eating response, not a logical one.

The person with intense cravings will resort to whatever will give them energy the quickest: sweets, chocolate, cake, bread, cookies, soft drinks and many other processed foods. These foods are quickly converted to sugar and blood-sugar levels rapidly rise. This will give the person immediate energy, but it will also cause the pancreas to produce the hormone insulin to regulate sugar levels in the blood. Insulin's job is to collect any excess sugar molecules and transition them out of the blood and into the cells.

Can you see the problem here? Insulin will try to get the unwanted sugar out of the blood and into the cells, however, the cell membranes are hardened and inflamed. Therefore, the sugar won't get absorbed, so it remains in the blood. Consequently, the pancreas releases more insulin in another attempt to lower blood-sugar levels. Again, its efforts to get the sugar through the cell membranes are blocked. This is a common condition called *insulin resistance*. If this situation continues in the body, the pancreas may finally get to a point where it stops producing insulin. Why would it continue to supply insulin if it's not doing the job? I'm sure you know what this is potentially leading to … yep, type II diabetes.

The scourge of the modern day, type II diabetes is growing rampantly out of control. In 2015, the International Diabetes Federation's *IDF Diabetes Atlas* estimated that:

- one in 11 adults has diabetes (415 million)
- one in two (47 per cent) adults with diabetes is undiagnosed
- 12 per cent of global health expenditure is spent on diabetes (US$673 billion)
- one in seven births is affected by gestational diabetes
- three-quarters of people with diabetes live in low- and middle-income countries
- every six seconds a person dies from diabetes (over five million deaths annually)

The most devastating statistic of all is that in most cases type II diabetes can be prevented, although it's currently being called an epidemic. Believe me, it's not an epidemic; it's a lifestyle choice. It's a choice you are making and can make each and every day. I've said it before and I'll say it again:

you are in control. When you start making different choices, you will start getting different results.

The great news is that your cell membranes are very sensitive to what you consume and therefore will be very responsive to any changes you make. It's a simple process: significantly reduce your omega-6 and trans fat consumption and increase your omega-3 intake. That means less bread, rice, pasta, biscuits, bakery products and processed foods. Surprise, surprise! It means more natural fruits, vegetables, quality proteins and the right fats. Surprise, surprise! It means a significant increase in your omega-3 consumption: more deep sea cold water fatty fish, flaxseed and leafy greens. Surprise, surprise!

I need to make a quick disclaimer here. If you are on medication for diabetes, please don't take it upon yourself to stop all medication. Certainly, start making the right changes with your eating and then sit down with a medical practitioner who is open to natural solutions and to working out a plan to transition you off medication and back to the optimal well-being you so rightfully deserve.

Nothing I've explained in the previous paragraphs is new or ground breaking. You know it, don't you? Maybe now with some extra knowledge and an understanding of the impact your eating is having on your cells, your well-being and your life, you might actually do something about it – there is a lot at stake.

Oh, my gosh, cell membranes are critical. I need you to pay close attention to the next thing I'm about to say. You may be eating lots of healthy foods, highly nutritious fruits and vegetables, you may even be taking a multivitamin/mineral supplement but still suffering from lethargy, fat gain, low immune system, inflammation and insulin resistance and wondering why. The reason is that you still haven't given your cell membranes what they need to be permeable enough to let those wonderful nutrients through and into the cells. In other words, much of those nutrients is being wasted if your omega-3 intake is insufficient.

The omega-3 to omega-6 ratio is the one you need to focus on. Think of it this way: omega-3 is the key that unlocks (softens) the cell membranes to allow the passage of those life-giving nutrients into the cells and power them up! Eat more fish and other sources of omega-3. In addition, I want to encourage you to source out and consume a quality omega-3 fish oil supplement. I take what many people consider an excessive number of quality fish oil capsules. Why? Because I find it difficult to eat enough quality natural sources of omega-3 and I need to look after my cell membranes – it's that simple.

The greatest challenge we have in consuming enough quality omega-3 to balance out the omega-3 to omega-6 ratio is as a result of limited options. To get enough omega-3 from plant sources would require eating an unrealistic amount of food. Please eat those foods; just don't expect that's all you need to do.

I've already mentioned that deep sea cold water fatty fish is possibly the best source of omega-3 fats. That's great, but how much fish are you eating and do you really know what you're eating? How has the fish been grown, what has it been fed and how has it been treated? The best sources are wild (not farmed) salmon, tuna, sardines, menhaden and anchovies. Honestly, when's the last time you ate any of those?

I'm not talking about the fish you get with your fish 'n' chips, I'm not talking about the canned fish you eat and I'm not even talking about the salmon you purchased at the market. I'm sure the reason why fish 'n' chips and canned fish are not great options is pretty obvious to you. The fish they use at the takeaway shops is rarely from the deep sea, and what they do to prepare that fish ruins any health benefits it may have. The processing required to get fish into a can will significantly compromise the quality and nutritional content of the fish.

You may, however, be questioning my comment about the salmon, so I'll answer that question with a short personal experience. A few years ago, Laura and I went to a fresh food market to buy the ingredients for a wonderfully fresh, tasty and healthy salmon dinner that evening. After we'd got all the vegetables we needed we went to the fresh fish counter. I asked the fishmonger whether the salmon was wild or farmed, and he laughed. That's not a good sign. He told me the fish was farmed and that getting wild fish would not be easy. I asked him the next obvious question: 'Where should I go to get wild salmon?' He looked at me with a serious look on his face and said, 'Canada!' Now, keep in mind I live in Melbourne, Australia, a long, long, long way from Canada.

'What's wrong with farmed fish?' I hear you asking. Good question. Do you remember what happened to chickens when demand for them grew? Closed confined cages, disgraceful conditions, low-quality synthetic feed, growth hormones to speed up the process, antibiotics to kill infections – all of which led to very unhappy chickens and dangerously unhealthy chicken meat. Fish farming has gone very much the same way.

Fish, and in particular salmon, are grown and harvested at high-speed rates in confined ponds. They are often fed synthetic food, which is a higher source of trans fat and omega-6. Understand what that means: the fish you are eating for its omega-3 properties is being fed largely from trans fat and omega-6 fat food sources. In other words, farmed salmon will have a lower content of omega-3 and higher content of omega-6 and trans fat. This is clearly not what we want.

In addition to this, consider that farmed salmon live in a very different environment to wild salmon, an environment that impacts the colour of the flesh. The beautiful dark pink colour we know and look for is common primarily to wild salmon. Because the rate at which farmers are causing the fish to grow, the flesh does not acquire the familiar pink colouring we know so well. How do you think suppliers of farmed salmon make their fish look wild? Yes: they artificially colour the flesh. Does this impact the quality of the fish? Does this change the taste? Will this have an effect on you if you eat it? I can't answer those questions; however, they are certainly worth reflecting on.

We live in a time when getting the best sources of food is more challenging than it's ever been, but it's not impossible. You are still able to make the right choices, and find the right foods and fats that will keep your cell membranes permeable enough to do what they need to do. You are still in control of the food you eat, the supplements you take and the nutrients you feed your body that allows your cells to do what they need to do to keep you optimally healthy.

Putting the pieces in place

I am a passionate and personally invested observer, as I've already mentioned. My goal for myself is to live a long, happy purpose-driven life and to share the things that I've seen, learned and experienced. For many years I suffered from severe eczema, which is a painful and irritating skin condition. It was itchy, it was annoying, it was ugly and it was all over my face and my body. I swallowed more pharmaceutical tablets, applied more cortisone cream and listened to more ideas that didn't work from the medical profession than I care to remember.

I finally started to investigate the condition and where it comes from. I discovered it's caused by chronic inflammation. I started to look at the things I was doing and the foods I was eating that may be contributing to this inflammation. I learned about what I've shared with you in this chapter and so I started making some changes that I'm about to recommend to you. I reduced the foods that were causing the inflammation and started significantly increasing my omega-3 intake.

I did eat more deep sea cold water fatty fish, even though it was farmed. I ate more leafy green vegetables and flaxseeds, even though I knew I couldn't eat enough. So I started supplementing with a quality omega-3 fish oil supplement, as I've also mentioned. Hear this, and hear this well: I suffered from eczema for most of my life with no remedy that I tried ever working, but within two weeks of making these changes my eczema was gone. Yes, I said gone, and it has never returned since I implemented these changes over 15 years ago.

Your cells are your units of life. They are powerful yet sensitive, they are responsive yet vulnerable. They are your responsibility to care for, so please do so. I urge you to take note of the action steps outlined below and get your cells doing for you what they are meant to do, so you can live the life you have the potential to live and be the person you were meant to be.

Key questions and action steps

1. Based on what you now know, how would you rate the health of your cell membranes and your cells' ability to be as effective as possible?

2. How do you feel about eating less processed food, that is, anything in a box, bag, tin or any other packaging?

3. How would you feel about buying less takeaway food and making your own healthier options?

4. Could you try to replace bread, rice and pasta with more fruits, salads and natural vegetables?

5. How do you feel about possibly eating more saturated fats and more grass-fed hens' eggs?

6. Would you be open to significantly increase your omega-3 intake: more deep sea cold water fatty fish, leafy green vegetables, flaxseed and walnuts?

7. Would you be open to supplementing with a high-quality fish oil capsule? That means one made with quality wild fish. I'll talk more about supplementation, what to look for and what to avoid, in the chapter 'Let food be thy medicine'.

8. Is your dream, your purpose and the important stuff in your life a strong enough motivator to make these changes?

5

The power of whole food
Go with your gut

… if Hippocrates was right and all disease does, in fact, begin in the gut, wouldn't that then mean that all healing and wellness will also begin in the gut?

Have you ever heard the saying 'go with your gut feeling'? Of course you have, and it is all about intuition. It's a powerful feeling coming from deep inside of you that wants to direct you towards and help you make decisions that align with your value system. It's quite possibly the most important feeling you can listen to, yet it's the one we most override and ignore, often regrettably. Do you know what I'm talking about? You have done it before, haven't you? You had a feeling in the pit of your stomach in response to a decision you'd made or were about to make yet you ignored it and made the decision anyway, right? How did it turn out? If you're anything like me, every time I've acted in conflict with my gut feeling it has ended badly. And I mean every time!

So, what does this actually have to do with the gut? Good question. Scientific studies are discovering that a key aspect of increasing mental sharpness and restoring or maintaining mental and emotional stability happens in the gut. It's even being referred to as your "second brain". Unknown to many, the gut is a very important organ when it comes to physical *and* mental and emotional health. The awareness that intestinal flora deficiencies are the root causes of a wide spectrum of immunity and mental problems is constantly expanding.

The gut is the object of much scorn, ridicule and negativity. We hate it when it gets bigger than we'd like it to be, even though it's because of our own decisions and habits that it grows. We blame it for bodily functions that can make our eyes water, our hair curl and our social life diminish, even though it's because of what we put in it that creates the issues. We hide it, we pierce it and we're often embarrassed by it. In this chapter, my goal is that you will learn to love it and treat it with the respect it deserves.

Our good friend Hippocrates said over 2,000 years ago: 'All disease begins in the gut.' Again, we didn't pay enough attention to this visionary man until very recently. In fact, research over the past two decades has revealed that gut health is critical to overall health and that an unhealthy gut contributes to a wide range of diseases, far more than just stomach pain, gas, bloating or diarrhoea. Gut imbalances have been linked to hormonal imbalances, auto-immune diseases, diabetes, obesity, rheumatoid arthritis, autism spectrum disorder, chronic fatigue, fibromyalgia, anxiety, depression, eczema, rosacea and many other chronic health problems.

Now, if Hippocrates was right and *all* disease does, in fact, begin in the gut, wouldn't that then mean that all healing and wellness will also begin in the gut? Many researchers believe that supporting intestinal health and restoring the integrity of the gut barrier will be the most important goals of well-being in the 21st century. There are two closely related variables that will determine our gut health: the **intestinal micro-organisms** (gut flora) and the **gut barrier**.

Get ready for some mind-blowing numbers. In the last chapter I mentioned that there are 37 trillion cells in the human body. Well, get this: in a space much smaller – contained within the human body – our gut is home to approximately 100,000,000,000,000, or 100 trillion, intestinal micro-organisms. It may be hard for you to comprehend the enormity of 100 trillion as a number so consider this: if you stacked 100 trillion dollar notes on top of each other they would rise 11 million kilometres (almost seven million miles), a distance equivalent to travelling from the earth to the moon and back more than 14 times.

Wow, that's an incredibly hard number of gut flora to comprehend. Try to picture this: if your intestines were taken out of your body, opened out and laid flat they would cover the entire surface of a tennis court, so to say they are critical for optimal wellness is the understatement of the year. Not only do gut flora deter invading pathogens or kill off some of the bad guys, they also signal other aspects of our immune system in other parts of our body. Gut flora promote normal gastrointestinal function, provide protection from infection, regulate metabolism and comprise more than 75 per cent of our immune system.

In terms of the relationship between friendly gut flora and pathogenic bacteria (the bad stuff), the scales need to be heavily lopsided. We need around 85 per cent good guys compared to 15 per cent bad guys. When it goes the other way, all sorts of physical and mental problems can arise. What would you imagine to be the greatest cause of all the issues arising from the gut? As we know, Hippocrates said: 'Let food be thy medicine and medicine by thy food.' What he may also have said in the case of the gut and gut flora in the 21st century is: 'We too often let food be thy poison and poison be thy food.'

There are three types of bacteria that make up the 100 trillion micro-organisms in the gut:

- **Beneficial**: these are the good guys. They help with the absorption of nutrients, give us energy, build our immune system, help us detoxify and maintain a healthy pH balance and the integrity of the gut barrier. We need at least 85 per cent of these wonderful super bacteria.
- **Pathogens**: these are the bad guys. They prevent absorption of nutrients, add toxicity to the body, break down the immune system,

impact pH balance, will steal your energy and contribute to leaky gut syndrome. We want to keep them below 15 per cent of the total.

- **Commensal**: these are the swingers and can go either way. They can become beneficial or they can become pathogenic, all depending on certain factors we can control.

Clearly, we want the commensal bacteria joining the good guys team, not the pathogenic team. This being the case it's vitally important to take control of the following potential stressors, which will push them to the dark side if we're not very deliberate.

I want to say before going any further that everything I write, everything you learn and everything you know will be of no help unless you take action to change your habits. Please don't just read this and say, 'Gee, that was interesting.' For your own sake – that of your health, your family, your life and everything that's important to you – take positive action TODAY!

Okay, that's off my chest. Let's discover how to go out and recruit the commensal bacteria to join the healthy gut flora team. There are certain stressors that will push these swinging voters over to the dark side; your job is to identify which apply to you and make the necessary changes. In fact, really your job is to just do what you know to do. Up until today, you may not be doing the things you know you should be doing. It's probably because you haven't yet connected your wellness to your 'why?' Today things will be different for you. Today is the day you stop putting off the important stuff and start working towards a long, happy, successful and healthy life. Below is a list of things to be wary of.

Medication: the majority of medications will shut down stomach acid production, which is the first step in the digestion process. What happens if we remove the first step? There can be no more steps, which can be devastating. Please take in carefully what I'm about to say: I believe there are natural and far more effective alternatives to the drugs you may be taking. Find someone who can help you put together a natural, holistic, sustainable and wellness-giving nutritional solution that will, over time, wean you off the medication. I do understand this may require some time and appropriate medical support. I'm certainly not suggesting you just stop taking medication without seeking wise and qualified counsel.

Refined sugar, carbohydrates and processed foods: these feed the pathogens and open the door for commensal bacteria to turn bad. One hundred years ago the average annual consumption of sugar by an individual was one to two kilograms (two to four pounds), whereas now it's more than 70 kilograms (154 pounds). You know what to do about this one, don't you? What were we eating 100 years ago? There is no shortage of information, evidence, advice and strategies; all that may be lacking is the one thing you have most control over, and that is taking positive action today!

Insufficient fermented foods: this will cause an imbalance in stomach acid production and therefore coax the commensal bacteria to the bad side. Fermented foods are wonderful for gut health as they raise stomach acids if they're too low and lower them if they're too high. How cool is that? Fermented foods include unpasteurised, unheated, salt-free cabbage, sauerkraut, pickles and other fermented vegetables such as kimchi. Raw milk and cheese will help if your stomach can handle it. Eating great prebiotic foods and getting your hands on a good-quality probiotic supplement are great ways to ensure you get enough for good gut health.

Antibiotics: these wipe out everything in the gut. Chiropractor and nutritionist Dr Justin Marchegiani DC describes it this way: if you take all of the plants out of a garden and then leave it alone, the first thing to grow back will be weeds. Antibiotics wipe out all the bacteria and leave the gut vulnerable to pathogens. My suggestion is to get help weaning you off any antibiotics and find some natural solutions to restoring good well-being. If you are coming off antibiotics deliberately, put good pre- and probiotics back into your gut.

The difference between pre- and probiotics can confuse people, including me. Let me try to help you understand the difference.

Prebiotic fibre is the *non-digestible part of foods* such as bananas, onions and garlic, Jerusalem artichokes, the skin of apples, chicory root, and beans. Prebiotic fibre goes through the small intestine undigested and is fermented when it reaches the large colon. This fermentation process feeds beneficial bacteria colonies (including probiotic bacteria) and helps to increase the number of desirable bacteria in our gut.

Probiotics are *live beneficial bacteria* that are naturally created by the process of fermentation in foods such as yoghurt, sauerkraut, miso soup, kimchi. Probiotics are also available in pill and powder form and as an added ingredient in products such as yoghurt and health drinks.

Chronic stress: this is a serious issue in the 21st century. I've already talked about this and will cover some nutritional solutions in Chapter 12. You should be aware that one of the impacts of chronic stress is that it throws the immune system out of balance. The immune system and gut health are intimately related, so everything you can do to reduce that stress on the body and mind will be instrumental in great gut health and overall optimal wellness. Purify your thinking, your environment, your air and your water. Purify your eating and follow all of the guidelines already discussed up to now and to be discussed in the proceeding chapters.

Chronic infections: these lower your stomach acids and enzyme production and consequently the effectiveness of your nutrition. You may have heard that you are what you eat. Wrong! In fact, you are what you eat, break down, absorb and assimilate. Reducing infection comes about by increasing the immune system to fight off the pathogens that cause the infection in the first place. In other words, we need to get those commensal bacteria on the right side of the fence. I think I've covered that in enough detail so far.

Dietary toxins: such as wheat and industrial seed oils. These attack the gut barrier and cause leaky gut syndrome, which is covered in more detail in the next section.

There are no shocks here, are there? As you can see, finding solutions and ways to have lots of the healthy gut flora you need is no real surprise, nor is it hard. It's doing the things you know you should be doing anyway. As I've asked you before and I'll ask again many times before you finish reading this book: are your dreams and purpose and values in life strong enough and important enough for you to make the changes you need to make? I'll talk later in the chapter about some specific ideas to maximise your healthy intestinal micro-organisms.

Looking after the gut barrier

I want to encourage you to now think about your gut or gastrointestinal tract. What is it really? It's basically a tube that runs from your mouth all the way to your anus, and I'm not talking about the planet! It includes the oesophagus, stomach, small and large intestines and, if taken out of the body, would stretch nine metres (30 feet). You may never have considered that while the contents of the gut run through the body, they are technically outside of the body. Anything that enters the mouth and is not digested will pass right out the other end. This is, in fact, one of the most important jobs of the gut – to keep foreign objects and toxins from entering the body.

Just as the key to a healthy cell is the cell membrane, the importance of the gut barrier is equally, if not more, critical to optimal well-being. The main difference is that while we actually *want* a semi-permeable cell membrane to allow the flow of nutrients in and the removal of waste products, we most definitely *do not want* a semi-permeable gut barrier. The sad reality is that for many people the intestinal barrier is attacked, breaks down and becomes permeable. This is seriously bad news, as it allows toxic waste that was never meant to enter the bloodstream and the body to penetrate and poison the body. This is called leaky gut syndrome, or intestinal permeability.

I'm so sick of talking about bad news, negative symptoms and poor health, and you must be sick of hearing about it. However, this is stuff we all need to know. Leaky gut syndrome is one of the main contributors to auto-immune problems affecting the skeletal system, the kidneys, the liver and the brain. In addition to this, leaky gut can manifest as skin problems such as eczema or psoriasis, heart failure, auto-immune conditions affecting the thyroid (Hashimoto's disease) or joints (rheumatoid arthritis), mental illness, autism spectrum disorder, depression and more. Interestingly, you don't need to have gut symptoms to be suffering from leaky gut.

Guess what causes it?

I know you're going to be shocked. I know you think it's just the luck of the draw. I know you think it's out of your control. Think again! As with just about any one of the modern-day wellness challenges, leaky gut syndrome is caused by poor nutrition, medication and stress. You can fix it and you can start today.

Researchers have identified a protein called zonulin that increases intestinal permeability. Zonulin production is increased through consumption of wheat- and gluten-containing foods such as bread, pasta and other processed grains. Other causes of leaky gut include the same things that destroy healthy gut flora: poor diet, medications (antibiotics, NSAIDs, steroids, antacids and so on), infections, stress, hormone imbalances and neurological conditions (brain trauma, stroke and neuro-degeneration).

Okay, enough of the depressing stuff; time for some solutions and an action plan. As always, the answers are simple. To effectively address these conditions, we must rebuild healthy gut flora and restore the integrity of our intestinal barrier.

Putting the pieces in place

Clearly the goal is to move to a far more natural way of eating, thinking, behaving and dealing with any gut health concerns. In this chapter we have discovered that medications can cause serious damage to the gut, and I have suggested more than once to look for natural solutions and get yourself off medication. Again, as I said previously, first seek advice from a qualified professional. What I will say, with the risk of ruffling some feathers, is that if you are dealing with a doctor who is unwilling to look at a more holistic and natural approach or who is not open to help you wean yourself off medication, then with all due respect find another doctor!

I want to share with you some really basic actions that will help you recruit those commensal bacteria to the beneficial side and significantly improve gut health so you can enjoy all the amazing benefits that go with it. In addition to the few suggestions I make, I would also recommend looking at YouTube videos and reading books, articles and blogs about good gut health. There are people out there far more knowledgeable and qualified than me.

I'm going to talk about things to *avoid or reduce* that are destroying desirable gut conditions and things to *include or implement* that will create a fabulous and life-giving gut environment. I want to encourage you to choose at least one thing *to avoid* and one thing *to add* to your weekly routine to start this wonderful process.

All of these are concepts you know and the ideas I've discussed throughout this chapter and the book. Now is that time to take what you know and turn it into what you do. Please commit to at least one action from each list and then, over time, aim to change all of these habits. Remember what Hippocrates said: 'All disease begins in the gut.' We, well at least I, therefore concluded all wellness must also begin in the gut.

These are things to *avoid or reduce* to put a halt to the disintegration of the gut bacteria and barrier:

- Stress: wow, this a big one, but steps can be taken today. Learn to breathe, do yoga, focus on what you're grateful for, find positive people to associate with, purify your water, purify your air and find your purpose.
- Rushing at meal times: slow down, chew your food, enjoy the taste and texture and be present at meal times.
- Sugar and processed foods: eat less added sugar, eat less bread, rice, pasta and all processed foods.

- Alcohol: alcohol causes inflammation in the gut. If alcohol is an issue for you, set a realistic goal for the next week, month and beyond. You know what that is, don't you?
- Highly processed and gluten-containing grains: find alternatives to the bread, biscuits, crackers, bakery items and grains included in this category. Which one/s could you eliminate?
- Medication: make an appointment with your practitioner to discuss the process of transitioning off medication, or find a practitioner open to helping you do this.

These are things to *include or implement* to ensure and improve the integrity of the gut bacteria and the barrier:

- Yoghurt: start eating a natural, full cream, pot-set yoghurt. Ensure it has no added sugars or artificial sweeteners. If you have a problem with dairy, try a natural and pure coconut yoghurt.
- Kefir: a fermented milk drink cultured from kefir grains.
- Kombucha: a slightly sour, lightly effervescent drink made with either a green or black tea base. Kombucha is produced by fermenting tea using a symbiotic colony of bacteria and yeast and is available ready to drink online and in good supermarkets and health food stores.
- Prebiotics and probiotics: add to the beneficial bacteria in the gut. Find a good-quality supplement to add to your daily regime.
- Fermented foods: unpasteurised, unheated, salt-free cabbage, sauerkraut, pickles and other fermented vegetables such as kimchi. Raw milk and cheese will help if your stomach can handle it.
- Omega-3: helps to replenish, recover and restore the gut lining. Add deep sea cold water fatty fish and a high-quality fish oil supplement.
- Beneficial fruits and vegetables: eat lots of leafy greens, and other beautifully fresh and natural fruits and vegetables in a variety of colours. Yummy!

Would you be willing to choose at least one action from each list and commit to creating a new habit? Then over time do you think it would be worth making gradual changes to create a healthy and happy gut environment? It all starts in your gut, which then impacts your health and will have an influence on your family and ultimately determine the quality of your life. Are you ready to prioritise your gut?

Key questions and action steps

1. Based on what you now know, how would you rate the health of your gut?

2. Does it worry you or excite you?

3. Are you clear on what you need to do to have a happy gut?

4. Why is it important for you to start taking positive action today to look after your one hundred trillion gut bacteria and your gut barrier?

5. Are you willing to commit to two positive actions today?

6. Make a list of the people you care about who you would like to influence to make better choices and have a healthy gut.

7. Do you truly understand your influence on the lives of these people?

8. Are you loving your gut now? Are you ready to go with your gut?

References/resources

https://www.mindbodygreen.com/0-14510/10-signs-you-have-an-unhealthy-gut-how-to-heal-it.html

https://chriskresser.com/9-steps-to-perfect-health-5-heal-your-gut/

https://branchbasics.com/ways-to-increase-stomach-acid-production/

'Boost and Fortify Your Second Brain', article by Paul Fassa, 19 May 2014, https://www.preventdisease.com/news/14/051914_Boost-Fortify-Second-Brain.shtml

Dr Justin Marchegiani DC, https://justinhealth.com

Donna Gates, https://bodyecology.com/articles

5

The power of whole food
Let food be thy medicine

*Please embed the attitude and understanding that only a
positive mind and nutrient-rich food can heal. No synthetic
alternative is a solution for optimal well-being.*

I can't help but keep coming back to my main man, Hippocrates. I think if
he was alive today we would be good friends and would go out for a fresh
juice or herbal tea regularly! This chapter is really about looking at nature and
food as your medicine. It's about truly understanding that you are in total
control of your wellness and your life. It's about getting excited and feeling
empowered to make the simple changes that will have an exponentially
positive impact on your life in many ways.

Well-known Australian cardiologist and author Dr Ross Walker started
challenging mainstream thinking and focusing on preventative cardiology
over 20 years ago. Before that time, as with many doctors, he went through
years of training and study that conditioned him to think a certain way about
diseases and the treatments of them. That approach didn't sit right with him

and now, via his speaking, books and online resources, he is impacting many lives through teaching a natural and preventative approach.

Dr Walker empowers people to think positively, eat nutrient-rich food, reduce stress, exercise regularly and take quality nutritional supplements. He jokes that he is putting himself, as a cardiologist, out of business! He is also very open to acknowledging the fact that he is not popular among many mainstream cardiologists for the same reason. Now his passion, his work is saving more lives than he did as a mainstream cardiologist. He is also significantly improving the quality of those lives as a result of his work. For more information about the great work Dr Ross Walker is doing, visit his website at: www.drrosswalker.com.

The reality is that there is a ridiculously disturbing amount of dis-ease all over the world and it's not improving through traditional means. In fact, it's getting worse with each day that passes. I truly respect the courage of people like Ross Walker, and his patients, to challenge the mainstream. He works with and helps his patients get off the medication that causes so many other issues and back to a more natural way of living. There are many inspiring stories out there, some I'll share and many others I'm sure you know about. These stories give us legitimate anecdotal evidence that food truly is thy medicine if we will allow medicine to be thy food.

Make no mistake about it: dis-ease is happening as a result of stress on the body. In the 21st century, stress is not an occasional happening, it's a chronic and an ongoing issue that needs to be addressed if optimal well-being is your aspiration. Hundreds of years ago when I was a lad life was simpler, and stress was really only the result of a few intermittent arguments with neighbours, running away from the occasional wild animals and the physical stress of a life without the help of modern technology.

In the 21st century, stress is the result of a hectic life and not enough time to do the things we want to and need to do. Stress is the consequence of less time with family and more time having to do things we don't love. Stress is part and parcel with this microwave, quick-fix, must-have-it-now society. Stress comes with the continual pursuit of making money and creating financial security and the ever-rising cost of living. Stress comes about through misunderstanding due to a lack of communication with other people. Stress affects us through the pollution in the air and the water and electromagnetic activity. Stress is thrust upon us every time we turn on the TV, flick on the radio, pick up the newspaper or spend time with negative and toxic people. Stress is consumed every time we eat processed or tampered-with food. Our body is stressed every time we do any sort of physical activity.

Can you see now that there is a good chance you and I are chronically stressed? Can you start to understand why your body is rebelling, reacting and revolting? Does it make sense that, through this stress and the impact on your mind and body, your physical well-being is threatened? Are you ready to take back control? Are you prepared to swim upstream of society and do what will give you the well-being and life you want? Are you ready to let food be thy medicine and medicine be thy food?

The great US football coach Vince Lombardi was a firm believer that the winning teams were the ones that were best at doing the fundamentals well. In fact, he would begin each football pre-season by getting his team together, holding up a football, and saying, 'Gentlemen, this is a football.' He would then go on to talk the team through the fundamentals of the game, even taking them out on the field to talk about the boundaries and the end zone, and that the goal was to get the football into the end zone.

Can you imagine how this was received by players? These were professional athletes who had played the game for years and were the best of the best. But Coach Lombardi's instincts proved to be spot on: over his nine years of coaching his team, the Green Bay Packers, finished third just *once* (his first year) and took home the championship five times. Why am I talking about football and Vince Lombardi? Because in any area of life including your health and well-being, fundamentals are critical.

Your body needs nutrients. There; I said it! You are probably reading this book and thinking: 'Of course, does this guy think I'm stupid?' No, I don't for one second think you're stupid. I do want to make sure you understand and are acting on the basic fundamentals. Your body requires nutrients of many varieties and in sufficient quantity for it to be able to function effectively and heal itself when required. The question you need to be asking yourself is: 'Am I giving myself all the nutrients I need for optimal well-being?'

You need macronutrients, micronutrients and phyto-nutrients. Macro-nutrients include proteins, fats and carbohydrates. Micronutrients include the many types of vitamins and minerals available, all of which are needed by your body for one reason or another. Phyto-nutrients include plant-based nutrients that have been shown to have beneficial properties and will be a large part of what contributes to your optimal wellness. For more specific information about these nutrients please refer to the many amazing resources that are available.

We are facing obvious health challenges in the 21st century (and beyond) for a couple of key reasons. First, the chronic stress we are facing physically breaks down our body and significantly increases our need for all types of nutrients. Second, the impact of the polluted environment on plants in addition to man's synthetic and chemical intervention critically reduces the nutrients that are now available from the food we eat. Can you see the problem? It's a simple mathematical formula: if you consume more of the nutrients you need for optimal health, you will be optimally healthy. If you eat less than you need your body is vulnerable to dis-ease, as we are seeing all over the world at rates that are disturbing to say the least.

I think it would be safe to say without too much fear of controversy that you probably need to be consuming more nutrients than you currently are. Agree? Therefore, the first step is to start eating a greater variety of natural foods, which will start to deliver these nutrients to your body. You might even consider researching the additional benefits of eating organically grown foods. You should absolutely look into supplementing your eating plan with high-quality and natural supplements. I will discuss this in more detail in the next chapter.

As a great starting point, aim to consume food from each of the five colour groups of fruits and vegetables: green, red, yellow/orange, white and purple. You should try and get each of the five colours in your day, every day; here's why:

- **Green** fruits and vegetables are great for cellular and vision health, strong bones and teeth and weight management. These foods include *kale, collard greens, spinach, green peppers, watercress, lettuce, zucchini, broccoli, Brussels sprouts, green beans, soybeans* and *green tea.*

- **Red** fruits and vegetables provide amazing anti-oxidant protection from chronic diseases. These foods include *red apples, cranberries, watermelon, pink grapefruit, guava, pomegranate, radishes, raspberries, strawberries, cherries* and *tomatoes.*

- **Yellow/orange** fruits and vegetables are great for eye health, healthy immune function, protecting antioxidants, healthy growth and development. These foods include *squash, papaya, corn, pineapple, lemons, passionfruit, oranges, rockmelon (cantaloupe), carrots, apricots, sweet potato* and *mandarins (tangerines).*

- **White** fruits and vegetables are great for maintaining healthy bones, circulatory health, supporting arterial function and weight management. These foods include *turnips, onions, mushrooms, horseradish, white kidney beans, parsnips, garlic, cauliflower, black-eyed peas* and *pears.*

- **Purple** fruits and vegetables are great for supporting vision and heart health and for anti-oxidant protection. These foods include *figs, grapes, blueberries, boysenberries, red cabbage, blackcurrants, eggplant, purple sweet potato, black beans, plums, beets* and *blackberries.*

You can see the amazing and wonderful variety you have to choose from. You don't need to force yourself to eat foods you dislike, but you do need to eat more colourful fruits and vegetables.

Will eating healthier and supplementing require an investment of time and money? Yes, it will. Will that be the thing that prevents you from prioritising the well-being of you and your family? I hope not. Here is some perspective and a guarantee: I promise you any time and money you invest now in creating optimal health will save you an incredible amount of time and money in the future. There is always a cost; my advice is to pay the cost now as an investment in terms of prevention, rather than down the track as you suffer and struggle to regain lost health.

Toxins be gone

The reality is that we are living in a toxic world. Toxins are everywhere and are entering our body at a staggering rate. Make no mistake about it: toxins are infiltrating, poisoning and breaking down your body. They are compromising your well-being and impacting every area of your life. The good news is that the solution is simple: reduce the toxins entering and impacting your body and eliminate the ones that are already there.

I have already spoken ad nauseam about sources of toxicity, but I'm going to hammer you with it again because you may not have been paying enough attention. *If you can eliminate a very high percentage of toxins by doing a few simple things, then why wouldn't you do them?* If in fact toxins are caused by the way we think, the things we do, the air we breathe, the water we drink and the food we eat, then the truth is we are largely responsible for toxicity on and in our body.

You may agree or disagree with that last statement, but either way I encourage you to consider the choices you are making every day. I assume no one forced you to think the worst, beat yourself up, watch the news, hang around negative people, have no direction in life, take things personally, react badly, stay working at a place you hate, watch TV when you could be improving yourself, eat the food you are eating, drink tap water, breathe polluted air in your home, focus on what you don't have, make excuses and the many other choices you are deliberately making.

If you agree that you control these thoughts and choices, then you can change any or all of these things right now. If you do, you will significantly reduce the toxins entering your body. Isn't that a good thing? Then all that's left is to eliminate any sneaky toxins that do get in, which is almost a full-time job for your body. It's hard work and it has a deteriorating effect on those organs responsible for elimination, such as the liver and kidneys. Do you want to help them out a bit?

When we think of how our body eliminates toxins, it's through one or more of its many openings. We sweat toxins through our pores. We propel toxins out of our nose when we blow or drip. We flood both emotional and chemical toxins out of our eye sockets when we cry. We expel toxins out of our mouth when we vomit. We urinate toxins out of you know where. When we sit down to 'drop the kids off at the pool' we eliminate toxins through our bowel. Each one of these bodily processes is critical as your body self-cleanses and detoxifies.

Oprah Winfrey had a daily ritual of crying to release any emotional and negative toxicity. So stop trying to be so strong and let the tears flow. The next time you have diarrhoea be happy that your body is eliminating toxins, so please don't take drugs to stop it. The next time you vomit, rejoice in the fact that your body is forcibly getting rid of dangerous toxins. Every time you have a runny nose, sweat, get acne or need to pee, get excited as your body knows what it's doing and is looking after you.

The question is, of all these avenues for eliminating which is the most effective and which can we help the most? Not long ago I was watching a short but incredibly powerful YouTube video by the well-known raw food and wellness evangelist David Wolfe. David was talking about detoxification and elimination and used the example of his cousin, who needed help losing weight.

I can't remember specifics, but his cousin was incredibly obese and unhealthy, weighing something like 160 kilograms (352 pounds). As you can imagine this guy was full of toxins, so David's first piece of advice to him was simple: start drinking two litres (67 fluid ounces) of purified water upon rising in the morning before putting anything else in his body.

Interestingly most people, including myself, assumed this would just result in a fuller bladder and more urination. So get this: on the first day his cousin lost more than six kilograms (13 pounds). This was all toxins that passed out of his bowel as a result of the water flushing it through. In an 18-month period he lost 68 kilograms (150 pounds), again largely toxins flushed out of his bowel and primarily because of the water he was drinking in the morning.

The bowel is the most effective path to quickly move toxins out of the body. All the other avenues will help, but they take too long. You want to get them out fast! Drinking one to two litres of purified water upon rising will ensure that those toxins are flushed through and eliminated. I've been doing this for the last two years and it works. In just the first six weeks I lost 14 centimetres (5.5 inches) from my gut. These were centimetres I didn't even know I had to lose!

I hope I have made this *simple step of removing toxins* clear enough. In addition to removing as many sources of toxins as you can, work towards drinking one to two litres of purified water every morning before anything else goes into your mouth. In answer to the question you may be asking yes, it must be purified water. If it's tap water it's not removing but adding toxins to the body.

Let's get radical

While you are deliberately doing all the right things to purify and detoxify, your body is also working away, 24/7, to destroy and keep any remaining toxins at bay. Inside your cells, chemical reactions are continually happening to remove and destroy toxins. The unfortunate by-products of these chemical reactions are nasty little atoms called **free radicals**.

I'm going to keep this as simple as possible. My main aim here is not that you have a full physiological and scientific understanding but that you understand the devastating impact of free radicals and commit to positive action. I hope you're okay with that.

The moment there is any stress on and toxicity in the body, chemical reactions start happening to eliminate the toxins. As mentioned, the by-product of these chemical reactions are free radicals – which are very unstable atoms missing an electron that react quickly with any other compounds to capture the needed electron and regain stability. When the attacked molecule loses an electron it becomes a free radical itself, and a chain reaction of damage begins. Once this process begins, it quickly escalates and results in the disruption of a living cell.

Some free radicals are produced normally during metabolism and are a part of the body's process to help neutralise viruses and bacteria. The body should be able to handle normal free radical activity, however, we live in crazy times. The chronic stress and pollution we are continually subjected to, in addition to the fact we are not eating enough of the nutrients that neutralise free radicals, mean they have become a seriously devastating problem.

I described already the multiplication and duplication of cells, that they will duplicate and multiply whatever state they are in. Disrupted or damaged cells will duplicate and multiply over time and cause dis-ease, illness and death. Yes, you heard me: many of the horrendous statistics of the modern-day ailments such as heart conditions and cancers are the result of free radical damage. Something needs to be done, and something needs to be done now by you and me!

I lost my mother to cancer and it was the most heartbreaking event of my life. She is only one of millions and millions of people impacted by a disease that can be prevented. I truly respect the people working tirelessly for cures, but I just wish more time, money and energy would be spent on prevention. We already have the cure, as Hippocrates said thousands of years ago. We just need to pay attention, take responsibility, be pro-active and stop being so reactive.

As I look back at my mother's cancer journey, I am continually inspired but also saddened. Her initial diagnosis of breast cancer was a shock, but looking back not a surprise. Her smoking, eating and emotional habits took her health down a free radical–forming path that, I believe, led to breast cancer. After this diagnosis, she took the conventional medical path and absolutely no responsibility. She went through a chemically, surgically and synthetically charged course of action to treat the symptoms, but made no effort to find and deal with the cause. Consequently, after 18 months of being told that the cancer was all gone and she was fine, it reared its ugly head again. This time it appeared in her liver, and this time the prognosis was not as optimistic.

My mother was given just a couple of years to live. She immediately changed her attitude and approach, deciding it was up to her to take control. The action she took, the changes she made, the life she then lived and the legacy she left inspire me every day. She turned a two- to three-year death sentence into a 16-year journey of joy, wellness and abundance. While she started on the wellness path later than she should and died younger than we all hoped, the things she did to change her circumstances are the same things we can all easily do, starting today.

The first thing she and my dad decided to do was to purify their environment. Surprise, surprise! My mother underwent hypnosis, started meditating, began a regime of positive affirmations, read positive books, attended inspiring and informative events and listened to empowering audios. Consequently, her mindset, self-esteem and attitude changed almost immediately. My mother and father installed water- and air-purification systems to stop the flow of toxins and development of free radicals. They even started to look at ways of reducing the electromagnetic radiation from all the gadgets, devices and electronics in the house. They started juicing and eating only natural and organic foods. They stopped eating red meat and only consumed the flesh of fish. One of the key things they did was to focus on consuming foods with a very high anti-oxidant content.

What is an anti-oxidant? Anti-oxidants are powerful properties of many different micro- and phyto-nutrients that neutralise free radicals. They do it by donating the electron and ending the electron-stealing reaction of the free radicals. The anti-oxidant nutrients themselves don't become free radicals after donating an electron because they are stable in either form. They act as scavengers, helping to prevent cell and tissue damage that could lead to cellular damage and disease.

Can you see where we're heading here? As always, work hard and make good choices to reduce and remove any source of toxins that could lead to free radical formation. Then, bombard your body with natural foods and natural supplements high in anti-oxidant properties. Again, it's a simple formula: if you have more anti-oxidants in your body than free radicals you're in great shape. If you have more free radicals than anti-oxidants in your body you are heading for disaster. How do you know? There are tests you can take to assess the free radical activity in your body, but my theory is you shouldn't give any free radicals a chance; let those anti-oxidants loose.

Vitamins A, C and E and many phyto-nutrients are high in anti-oxidants and what you want to be consuming. Eat lots of leafy greens including kale and spinach (Popeye can't be wrong!). Get into sprouts, like Brussels and alfalfa, which are a fabulous source of anti-oxidants. I used to joke that no one could possibly enjoy Brussels sprouts and now they are one of my favourite foods. Enjoy a wide variety of different coloured vegetables, including beets, broccoli, corn, eggplant, onions and red capsicums (bell peppers) to colour up your plate. Enjoy eating some delicious fruits, including berries, cherries, grapes, plums and oranges. Teas of many varieties, particularly herbal teas, are a very high source of anti-oxidants.

If you're like many people, including myself, you're looking at that list of foods thinking: great, what about the taste? Here is the same answer I'm going to give you that was provided to me one day as I was listening to an audio. The speaker was talking about her daughter, who was never really into the whole healthy fruits and vegetables thing. One day as her mother served her up a yummy plate full of vegetables her reaction was, 'Oh, do I have to? These vegetables taste so bland!' Her mother looked at her and responded, 'Sometimes there has to be a purpose greater than taste.'

Get excited about the taste of filling your body with anti-oxidants. Get passionate about the taste of feeling healthy. Enjoy the taste of looking lean and fabulous. There's something empowering about the taste of making good choices. Can you imagine the relieving taste of restoring lost health? The taste is there if you can focus on the benefits, the rewards and the optimal health it's leading you towards.

Now, if that's not enough, here's some great news: dark chocolate and red wine are both powerful anti-oxidants. This was exciting news for me when I found out about it. In fact, one study shows that dark chocolate has higher anti-oxidant activity than blueberries, which were for a long time considered the highest of anti-oxidant–rich foods. Red wine contains different types of flavonoids, which are very powerful anti-oxidants.

The obvious condition on chocolate and wine consumption is this: don't get carried away. The dark chocolate must be high quality, organic if possible, and at least 70 per cent cocoa content; just one to two squares per day will have amazing wellness benefits. I said one to two squares, not one to two blocks. A small glass of good-quality red wine every day or every second day will give you wonderful wellness benefits. I said one glass per day, not one bottle. Enjoy your chocolate and wine in moderation along with the wellness benefits that come with them.

Free radicals are only an issue if they are allowed to run riot. You are in total control here – yes, you are! You get to choose the things you can do, as I've suggested, to reduce stress and toxicity in the body and you're the one who decides what you put in your mouth. Just before you take that next bite of whatever it is you are tempted to eat, ask yourself: is this going to take me towards optimal health and longevity, or take me towards a place where I definitely do not want to end up?

Controlling cortisol

Back in prehistoric times, if you can imagine, life was much simpler. Among the cave people community there was a man named Ugg and his woman Igg. Ugg loved Igg and would take her with him everywhere he went, dragging her along the ground by her hair. Life was great, as they lived simply and enjoyed everything that nature had to offer: sun, open spaces, fresh food, pure air and clean water. There were only occasional challenges, those rare instances when Ugg had to avoid the clutches of the devilish *Tyrannosaurus rex*.

One day, Ugg strolled out of his cave to do some berry picking, when a few minutes later he heard that terrifyingly unmistakable sound behind him. It was the nasal snorting of *T. rex*. He turned slowly, heart racing, to see those fearsome eyes staring straight at him and a hungry *T. rex* drooling over his next meal. Ugg had other plans. He felt the hormones and emotions build in his body, and he felt himself growing a bit taller as he prepared himself for drastic action.

He looked at *T. rex*, screamed at the top of his lungs and turned and ran in the opposite direction as fast as he could. From somewhere within he found the speed and agility he didn't know he had as he darted in and around trees, over hills and through caves with *T. rex* hungry and hot on his tail. There were a few close calls and *T. rex* almost had his dinner, but somehow Ugg evaded the beast, found his way back to his cave, slammed the rock door behind and collapsed at the feet of Igg. He was safe at last! Ugg spent the next 30 minutes recovering his gasping breath, allowing his heart rate to return to normal and enjoying it as his fear and anxiety melted away.

What was it that saved Ugg from the *T. rex*? Among other things, it was cortisol. Cortisol is a steroid hormone that is produced by the adrenal glands and released when there is any stress on or perceived threat to the body. It's a 'fight or flight' hormone. It worked beautifully for me in my days as a professional footballer; any time there was an angry opposition player heading for me I was very grateful for cortisol. I used to joke – even though I wasn't joking when I said it – I won all of my fights by 50 metres!

In Ugg's case, the moment he was aware of *T. rex* and his imminent danger, his adrenal glands responded by releasing cortisol into the bloodstream. The result was that his blood sugar levels rose and his blood pressure increased in preparation for him to stand and fight or to turn and run. It was a good thing for Ugg he took the latter option: it gave him speed, strength and agility that he didn't know he had and it enabled him to escape the clutches of the fierce beast and get safely back to his cave. After a short period of time his body stopped producing cortisol, his blood sugar and blood pressure levels returned to normal and all was good. Ugg and Igg just had to eat leftovers that night because Ugg was unable to collect any fresh berries.

As you can see from that story, cortisol is a good thing and is necessary for all of us at times in our life. When stress and danger are occasional things, cortisol is useful and a very important bodily function for all of us. Let's fast forward the tape from the prehistoric age to today: is stress an occasional thing, or is it a chronic and ongoing issue? I think you know the answer to that.

According to physician and speaker Dr Lissa Rankin MD, our bodies know how to heal themselves. In her new book *Mind Over Medicine: Scientific proof that you can heal yourself* she shares data about the placebo effect, which provides concrete proof the body is equipped with natural self-repair mechanisms that are under the control of our brilliant minds. Our bodies know how to fix broken proteins, kill cancer cells, retard aging, and fight infection. They even know how to heal ulcers, make skin lesions disappear and knit together broken bones. The problem is that the self-repair mechanisms don't work if you're stressed.

With all of the stress on our body – which I have talked about too much already – the body is over-producing cortisol, which is proving to be a serious issue. Dr Rankin lists ten signs that cortisol is being over-produced in your body:

- *Sleep is affected* due to high cortisol levels, which should drop at night to allow your body to relax and recharge. However, chronically high cortisol levels can cause a second wind right around bedtime, making sleep more challenging.

- *Feeling fatigued, even with proper sleep.* Over time, high levels of cortisol deplete the adrenal glands and predispose you to chronic fatigue.

- *Weight gain, especially around your abdomen, even when you eat well and exercise.* Cortisol causes an increase in blood sugar, which can make you thick around the middle even when you're doing everything right.

- *More susceptibility to colds and other infections.* Cortisol de-activates your body's natural self-repair mechanisms, in turn affecting your immune system, leaving you vulnerable to infection and illness.

- *Unhealthy craving*, because cortisol raises your blood sugar levels, thus increasing the risk of diabetes. It also causes an increased production of insulin levels, leading to a drop in blood sugar, feelings of lethargy and the predictable craving that comes with it.

- *More prone to backaches and headaches.* As mentioned, chronically high cortisol levels deplete your adrenal glands, which raises prolactin levels, increasing the body's sensitivity to pain such as backaches and muscle aches. Excessive cortisol also creates an excessive sensitivity in the brain to any pain, which means that even the slightest twinge can activate the nerves of the brain, causing headaches.

- *Sex drive is diminished.* When stress hormones are high, libido-inducing hormones such as testosterone drop. That is not good news for anyone!

- *Gut issues.* Your gastrointestinal system is very sensitive to stress hormones such as cortisol. Nausea, heartburn, abdominal cramps, diarrhoea or constipation can result from excessive stress hormones.

- *Feeling anxious.* High levels of cortisol and adrenaline can lead to jitters, nervousness, anxiety, feelings of panic and even paranoia.

- *Mood swings.* High levels of cortisol suppress the production of serotonin, which is the hormone in the body responsible for mood balance. A deficiency can lead to negative thoughts and even depression.

Clearly, cortisol is not a good thing when there's too much of it, so how do we keep it to a healthy and beneficial level? I'm glad you asked. I'm sure if I tell you one more time to reduce stress on the body – by thinking better, focusing on your purpose, finding positive people to associate with, forgiving yourself and others, listening to positive audios, reading uplifting books, watching less TV and news, purifying your air and water, eating less processed and tampered-with food – I believe you may burn this book. So I won't mention it again!

I do want to encourage you to do some research on an incredible herb by the name of *Rhodiola rosea*. As always I'm going to give you a layman's explanation, but you should know it's an amazing herb with many benefits including strengthening the nervous system, fighting depression, enhancing immunity, elevating the capacity for exercise, enhancing memory, aiding weight reduction, increasing sexual function and improving energy levels. If you look at the negative effects of cortisol, you will see that *Rhodiola* seems to effectively counter pretty much all of them. How?

Rhodiola is what's called an adaptogenic herb, which simply means that it's like a thermostat. In other words, it's released by the body when needed to regulate cortisol. One of the unique properties of this super herb is that, unlike water-soluble vitamins that the body won't store if not needed, *Rhodiola* is held by the body and released when required. So when energy is lacking and a lift is required the body releases *Rhodiola* to help with focus and stamina. In times of stress, anxiety and trauma, when the body responds by over-producing cortisol, again *Rhodiola* is released to regulate the cortisol and its negative impact on the body. Two randomised, double-blind, placebo-controlled trials of the standardised extract of *Rhodiola rosea* root provide a degree of support for these claimed adaptogenic properties.

I experienced the true power and value of *Rhodiola* a few years ago. My wife Laura and I, after many years of unsuccessful attempts, reluctantly decided to give IVF a try in order to have a baby. If you know anything about IVF you will know how stressful it is, particularly for the woman. Laura had to inject medication into her stomach every day for many weeks, while I watched, supported and almost passed out each time. The end result of two expensive cycles was no child and a very toxic wife.

The drugs in Laura's body created incredible stress and, as a result, she put on a significant amount of weight around her middle. We can only assume it was the impact of increased cortisol. She tried many things to lose the weight, all normal stuff such as eating better, exercising and trying to relax as much as possible. None had any real effect. Guess what did? She started taking two *Rhodiola* organically grown plant-based tablets each morning, and within just a few weeks the fat around her middle was as good as gone. Hallelujah to *Rhodiola*!

Time for a breath

Wow, I've just looked back over this chapter. It's longer than I thought it would be and I still have lots to talk about, so let's reconvene in the next chapter and continue this important subject of allowing nature to provide all the energy, medicine and abundance you need for amazing well-being.

Putting the pieces in place

Food, food, food: eat it and enjoy it. Eat real food, natural food, organic food, nutrient-dense food, a variety of coloured vegetables and fruits and foods that you honestly know you should be eating, right? Again, I come back to your 'why?' The great motivational speaker Jim Rohn said: 'Take care of your body, it's the only place you have to live.' Is he right, or is he right? He's right, all right! The question is not whether or not Jim Rohn is correct; the question is: are you ready to take positive steps to protect your home?

If so, then this chapter has reinforced the need to fill your body full of quality nutrients to ensure it can cope with any toxicity or stress that will surely challenge it. Please embed the attitude and understanding that only a positive mind and nutrient-rich food can heal. There are no synthetic alternatives as a solution for optimal well-being.

Are you ready to saturate your body with life-giving, healing and energy-producing food? Great!

Key questions and action steps

1. Honestly assess your nutritional intake and ask yourself this question: if I continue to eat what and how I'm eating today, how will my health be in one year, five years, 10 years and beyond? Will you be healthy? Will you still be around? Are you ready to do something?

2. How would you rate your level of toxicity? What steps could you take to reduce toxins entering your body?

3. Would you be willing to try drinking at least one litre (34 fluid ounces) of purified water every morning before any other consumption to help flush any remaining toxins out of your body?

4. Are you concerned about free radical activity in your body?

5. If so, are you ready to reduce stress and toxicity in your body as much as possible? What foods or natural supplements, high in anti-oxidants, would you be prepared to start consuming?

6. Do you think cortisol is affecting your body and your health? If so, are you ready to reduce stress and toxicity in your body as much as possible?

7. Source out a high-quality and natural *Rhodiola* supplement and take it as prescribed. Contact me if you have trouble sourcing it.

8. Aim to consume at least five different-coloured fruits and vegetables each day: white, green, orange, red, purple. Each colour will have a unique and very positive benefit on your well-being.

References/resources

www.healthchecksystems.com

https://authoritynutrition.com/7-health-benefits-dark-chocolate http://www.frenchscout.com/polyphenols

https://www.livestrong.com/article/410646-how-to-fast-before-test-for-cortisol-levels/

http://lissarankin.com/10-signs-you-have-way-too-much-cortisol

https://www.medicalnewstoday.com/kc/serotonin-facts-232248

https://www.herbwisdom.com/herb-rhodiola.html

5

The power of whole food
Nature provides everything we need

The people who are optimally healthy, focus on each and every decision, each and every day. They focus on good choices, good attitudes and what they can have rather than what they can't.

If you remember, I've spoken several times earlier in the book about Sherry Strong's nature principle. There are three very powerful and profound aspects of this principle I want to reinforce with you now. Again, I want you to be very clear that nothing I'm writing in this book is new, nor is it purely mine. I'm a messenger, not the message! Please clearly understand these three parts to the nature principle:

1. Nature provides everything we need for optimal well-being.
2. The more readily available a nutrient is in nature, the more we need to consume it.
3. When choosing food to eat and nutrients to consume, the healthiest options are those most easily obtained in nature.

Principle 1 really doesn't need much detailed analysis, does it? I think we can all agree with that one. Principle 2 I've spoken about, and we know the two most abundant nutrients on the planet are the ones we tend to think least about: air and water. There is one other nutrient that is abundantly and readily available in nature, yet most people are significantly deficient in it: stay tuned. Principle 3 needs to be in the front of our mind with many of the decisions we make during our day. I'm going to discuss some ways we can get even more out of nature and our food in this chapter.

Don't waste nature's greatest source of life

Imagine a world with no sun. Unimaginable, isn't it? Do you know why? There can be no life on earth, or probably any other planet without the sun. Among many things the sun provides light, warmth, energy – which helps plants photosynthesise – and rays which, when in contact with the human skin, facilitate production of the critical nutrient vitamin D.

If we look at the second of the nature principles, it states: the more abundant a nutrient is in nature, the more we need it for optimal well-being. Where would you think sunlight and Vitamin D sit? The sun is always there and the sun is free and readily available, and it's by far the best source of vitamin D.

Vitamin D deficiency should never happen, but it does for many people and it's causing serious issues including depression, schizophrenia, Alzheimer's, heart disease, high blood pressure, muscle aches and weakness, Crohn's disease, MS, rheumatoid arthritis, asthma, type I diabetes, rickets, osteoporosis, cancer, influenza and tuberculosis, just to name a few.

It's crazy to think we may be suffering from one of these conditions when the solution can be as simple as allowing five to 10 minutes of direct skin exposure to the sun just two to three days per week. In winter, when there is not as much sun, it is not hard to choose some nutritional sources of vitamin D such as fish oils, fatty fish, mushrooms, beef liver, cheese, egg yolks and a good-quality supplement.

Let's get back to our good friend the sun. Why does it get such a bad rap, and why are we so afraid of any exposure to it? We have been so conditioned, over so many years, to believe that exposure to the sun is a bad thing that will lead to skin problems and cancers, and that it's easier to avoid it than take any risks. Advertisements on television and the horrendous images they portray of the effects of skin cancer and the impact on families are meant to scare us. And it's working for many people, to their own personal detriment. Fear is stopping people going outside, for even a short time, without covering every square inch of their bodies.

Don't misunderstand what I'm saying here: to go outside in the sun unprotected for many hours on end is a recipe for disaster and may very well end badly. However, you need sunlight and you need sunlight on unprotected skin for short periods of time, on a regular basis. You need sunlight, your children need sunlight and we all need sunlight. We need it because our body produces our own vitamin D3 when the skin is exposed to the sun's ultraviolet rays, specifically the ultraviolet (UVB) radiation. When UVB rays hit our skin, a chemical reaction happens. This chemical reaction begins the process of converting a prohormone in the skin into vitamin D. If I get into any more detail I'll confuse both you and me!

Many studies seem to indicate that, to allow the body to produce all the vitamin D it needs, the appropriate exposure is five to 30 minutes on your unprotected face, arms, legs and back between the hours of 10 am and 3 pm two to three times per week; the timing will depend on skin type and sensitivity. Your body is such an amazing blessing and is ready, willing and able to help you, heal you and hone you if you give it the raw materials it needs. Sunlight on unprotected bare skin is one of those raw materials it needs on a regular basis.

Yes, the sun can burn and be harmful. Yes, the impact of global warming in modern times has changed things. Yes, there are times when you do need to cover up and reduce over-exposure to the sun. Be smart about protecting yourself and be very wary of anything you are applying to your body. Do you know that any cream or liquid you apply to your skin will be absorbed through the porous skin and into the bloodstream? Do you use a sunscreen regularly? Do you know what's in that sunscreen? Is it chemical or natural? What impact will it have on toxicity, free radical and cortisol activity in the body? These are questions to consider carefully.

Can I suggest that you very much limit sunscreen and, when the time is appropriate, cover yourself up with hats, long-sleeved tops and long pants? In addition to wearing more clothes, there are some great sun block alternatives:

- *Eat well.* Surprise, surprise: eating foods rich in healthy fats and anti-oxidants helps protect your skin from damage, including UV damage. In fact, well-known Australian naturopath Bec Farah wrote an article in the February 2017 issue of *LivingNow* magazine called 'Eat your sunscreen'. She discussed the properties of certain foods to block harmful UV rays, repair damaged skin and to protect us from the negative effects of the sun. These foods include aloe vera, green tea, almonds, grapes, pomegranate, tomatoes, cucumber and cruciferous vegetables such as broccoli, cabbage, Brussels sprouts, turnips, cauliflower and radishes. In addition to this, dark, colourful fruits and vegetables contain carotenoids and other powerful anti-oxidants. Carotenoids give your skin a healthy bronze glow even without sunlight while making sure you burn less often. Nuts, seeds, coconut oil, avocados, sea vegetables, micro-algae and even some healthy saturated fats have also been shown to be beneficial.

- *Astaxanthin.* This anti-oxidant is also a carotenoid and gives salmon their reddish pink colouring. The salmon get it from micro-algae that produce astaxanthin, and it protects themselves from UV rays. Astaxanthin is more powerful than vitamin C, vitamin E or CoQ10 (an anti-oxidant). It protects our skin from solar injuries and even helps prevent DNA from being damaged by ultraviolet rays. It is literally a bit of sunscreen in a pill, but it also protects the heart, brain, joints and eyes.

- *Red raspberry seed oil.* This is one of the best seed-oil sunscreens. It averages between 28 to 50 SPF and blocks troublesome UVB rays.

- *Carrot seed oil.* Carrot seed oil may be a little harder to find, but it has 38 to 50 SPF and is high in carotenoid anti-oxidants.

- *Wheatgerm oil.* Wheatgerm oil is a great moisturiser but also has an SPF of twenty.

- *Sesame oil.* Sesame oil blocks 30 per cent of sunlight, letting you stay in the sun longer without burning. Apply it every hour or two if you plan to be out longer.

- *Coconut oil.* Coconut oil blocks about 20 per cent of the sun's rays. It also moisturises skin, lessens inflammation and smooths out blemishes while it limits solar damage. Coconut oil works even more if you take it internally. It fights inflammation from the inside and contributes to the healthy production of vitamin D.

- *Aloe vera.* Aloe vera is often used on a sunburn to soothe hot, burned skin. It works beforehand too by blocking out about 20 per cent of sunlight.

- *Natural sunscreens.* Check the labels and understand the impact of any ingredient you are putting on your skin.

Food: a wonderful joy and powerful preventative

One of my previous books was based primarily on the *if–then* premise, that *if* we have to eat to live *then* why not enjoy it? Almost 30 years in the personal training and wellness industry has illustrated to me that far too many people lose sight of the 'enjoyment factor' as they obsessively pursue a look they will probably never maintain. I've seen people diet, sacrifice, starve and willpower themselves into oblivion by focusing on the wrong things.

They focus on the scales, the tape measure, the mirror; in other words, the result! Consequently, any slight variation in the wrong direction sends them spiralling off into a place from which many never recover. As a footballer playing in a losing team for many years, I learned that when we continually focused on the scoreboard and who was winning or losing, we continually lost! When I moved from a football club with a loser's mindset to one with a winner's mindset, the focus was totally different. The winning team focused on the right training, the right attitudes, the right skills, the right actions and the right habits. As a result, the scoreboard took care of itself and we won far more than we lost.

Those who yo-yo diet and jump from one gym to another, one wellness plan to another and one eating plan to the next are focused on the results. They erroneously believe anything that doesn't give them immediate results isn't working. So they continually stop, start and ultimately fail through frustration and disappointment. That sounds like no fun to me.

The people who are optimally healthy, who look and feel amazing and who love the process focus on each and every decision, each and every day. They focus on good choices, they focus on good attitudes and they focus on what they can have rather than what they can't. They love the amazing array of delicious fresh foods available for them to choose from and they enjoy the feeling of putting those nutrient-rich foods in their body. They know that any indulgence they enjoy, in moderation, will not be detrimental to their well-being; instead it will be incredibly enjoyable and beneficial.

When these people choose to indulge, they do it at a time when they are feeling great and in full control of healthy choices. They are not indulging as the result of emotional turmoil or a powerful and dangerous craving, which takes hold of many people. I will discuss this critical area in more detail in the next chapter. Eating the right foods at the right time of the day and making better lifestyle choices, as I've already discussed in earlier chapters, will enable you to get to this place in your own life.

The question now arises around the 'right foods' and whether they really do still have the nutritional content they had back when Ugg was a boy. Debates are raging as to whether organically grown foods are better than traditionally grown foods, and whether nutritional supplements are effective and necessary or just expensive urine. These are decisions you are going to need to make for yourself, just as I did.

Amazing Angela

A good friend of mine, Greg, has a background as a carpenter and currently works in the live theatre industry. He is not a wellness professional. He is, however, someone who committed himself to his own well-being many years ago and is now someone I would consider more knowledgeable about long-term wellness than many. Greg and his siblings have recently helped their 82-year-old mother, Angela, to a new beginning and a renewed lease on life.

The following story is as it was told to me by Greg. I truly respect Greg and his siblings for the courage they showed to challenge conventional medical thinking. I have total admiration for Angela, who has decided she's not too old to live her life to the fullest. I'm inspired by this and I'm excited to share it, and I hope it impacts you as it has me.

At age 60 Angela, who had been going through some turmoil in her life, was feeling a bit down emotionally, so went to see her doctor to try to get some answers for the way she was feeling. With only the best intentions, but not much analysis, she was prescribed an anti-depressant medication. One of the side effects of this medication was high blood pressure, which quickly developed. Consequently, Angela was then put on a blood-pressure medication to control this imbalance. Crazy: a drug to deal with side effects of another drug!

If that wasn't bad enough, over time drowsiness and dizziness developed as a side effect of both medications combined, so guess what? Yes, another drug, an anti-psychotic, was prescribed. Despite not drinking alcohol or eating anything containing sugar, and having what most would consider a very healthy diet and lifestyle, wellness was now a struggle for Angela. The dizziness continued to get worse to the point that, in her late 70s, she was diagnosed with a neurological condition that was suspected to be partly due to long-term use of the brain chemistry-altering medications Angela was taking. She was trialled on various drugs to help, but insanely ended up back on the three original medications.

Shortly after her 81st birthday Angela became very ill and was rushed to hospital, vomiting and semi-conscious. She was taken off medications until her consciousness returned and was then placed on a drip, until gradually she recovered. A few weeks after getting home from the hospital the same episode repeated itself, and again she was treated the same way. She eventually returned home. A few weeks later, in December 2016, she was again rushed to the hospital and this time the symptoms were even more severe. A very observant doctor in emergency ran a series of tests and concluded that the combination of medications was causing severe hyponatremia. This condition is defined at https://www.mayoclinic.org thus:

> Hyponatremia occurs when the concentration of sodium in your blood is abnormally low. Sodium is an electrolyte, and it helps regulate the amount of water that's in and around your cells.
>
> In hyponatremia, one or more factors – ranging from an underlying medical condition to drinking too much water – cause the sodium in your body to become diluted. When this happens, your body's water levels rise, and your cells begin to swell. This swelling can cause many health problems, from mild to life-threatening.

Greg and his siblings, who had power of attorney, decided it was time to take control of their mother's well-being. They insisted she not be given any drug unless it was necessary for her life. As an alternative, they supplied the hospital with high-quality omega-3 capsules to improve Angela's cell membranes, organic plant-based multivitamins for enhanced nutrition and *Rhodiola* tablets to replace the anti-depressants. As you can imagine, this initiative was met with opposition from several conventionally trained doctors, but because of the courage and strength of conviction of Angela's children it was eventually agreed upon.

Angela detoxified in hospital with the organic supplements and was taken off all her medications, and the results were mind blowing. Her blood pressure was perfect without medication and her intellectual awareness returned to what it had been like many years earlier, in fact, back to the time before she was initially prescribed anti-depressants. At the end of January 2017, Angela was living independently and was on zero medications. Her nutritional supplements included multivitamins, omega-3, *Rhodiola*, milk thistle and dandelion, *Ginkgo biloba*, valerian, and cranberry and garlic supplements. Wherever possible, they are organically-grown plant based supplements. She is now reading affirmations daily, listening to positive mindset audios and has a new purpose for living. Angela is loving life and is totally drug free!

I love this story and I loved sharing it. I hope it inspires you as much as it did me. It again highlights the power of the right thinking and the right association and the ingestion of organically grown food and supplements.

Let's talk about these two hotly debated topics: organically grown food and nutritional supplements. I don't know about you, but I want to stack the odds in my favour. I don't want to leave anything to chance or to wait until a double-blinded study finally provides the evidence of what we intuitively know already, that organically grown food is a far better option for optimal well-being. If you talk to different people you will get many different opinions. Most people believe they are giving you good sound advice. However, what they are actually giving is mainly just 'sound' and very little 'good advice'!

For what it's worth, I'm of the opinion that if there's a chance that organically grown food has a higher nutrient content and less chemicals and will get me closer to optimal health – and there is a very good chance – then, I'm going to eat it. It's certainly not going to do me any harm. Rather than go into details and reasons as to why you should eat organically grown foods, I want to recommend you just do it. Why? Because, if you've got this far into the book and optimal wellness is your aim, then there really is no other choice.

One thing I will say, when looking for organically grown foods, is to make sure they are certified organic. Joe Bloggs down the road may tell you he is growing organic fruits and vegetables in his garden, but he's probably kidding himself. The local greengrocer may declare that his produce is organic, but make sure you ask the right questions. Unless the land has been certified by a governing body stating that the soil is chemical free and full of the necessary micro-organisms and nutrients, only natural pest-control strategies are employed, purified water is used and all surrounding properties are chemical free, it's not organic!

Organic simply means 'as nature intended'. Anything that influences, impacts and affects the food that is not as nature intended will compromise its quality and add toxicity, and that impact will be passed on to you when you eat it. Look for certification every time for both natural foods and plant-based nutritional supplements.

To supplement or not to supplement? That is the question

You've just read Angela's story, which said most of what I wanted to say in a compelling way. I just want to encourage you to use your logical mind for a moment and satisfy yourself with the answer to these questions:

- Would you consider the food you eat today, based on the way it is processed, produced, farmed, handled, stored and treated, to have all of the nutrients you currently require for optimal well-being?

- Do you currently eat enough of the naturally nutrient-rich foods to give yourself the chance of getting all the nutrients you need for optimal well-being?

- Do you think that the impact of stress and toxins on your body, as discussed throughout this book, has created a need for an increased amount of daily nutrients than was required years ago?

- If you knew that being on a regime of quality food supplements would increase your nutrient intake, fill any nutritional deficiencies and enhance your physical and mental well-being, would you be willing to invest?

- Based on positive answers to the above questions, if you're not currently taking any food supplements then what is stopping you?

There could be several answers to the last question. Maybe justifying the extra cost is a challenge for you. Perhaps you're confused because there are so many choices and you are unsure which are the best products to choose. It may be that you are of the belief that vitamins are expensive urine and a waste of money. Or it could be something else that seems to you a valid reason as to why you're resisting this decision.

I want to deal with some of your concerns, but I think the best place to start – before even thinking about what type or brand of supplement – is to truly believe that you need to take them. Not as a replacement for real food but, as the name indicates, as a supplement to good eating habits. In the June 2002 issue of the *Journal of the American Medical Association*, it stated: 'We are eating enough to prevent deficiency, but not enough to prevent disease. We recommend that all adults take a multi-vitamin daily.'

This was recommended back in 2002, seventeen years ago. Do you think there is a greater need for nutrients today than there was back then? Why don't you try to decide that for yourself. The following questions are for you to assess your current lifestyle and personal and nutritional profile to help you decide whether you do actually need to supplement. It's simple: if you answer 'yes' to any one or more of the following, you will absolutely benefit from a quality supplement:

- Do you need more energy?
- Do you feel tired or run down at times?
- Do you crave sweet food?
- Do you have trouble losing fat?
- Do you eat less than nine serves of fruits and vegetables per day?
- Do you consume less than four serves of wild deep sea fatty fish per week?
- Do you eat mainly non-organic foods?
- Do you ever eat processed foods?

- Do you consume more than four alcoholic drinks weekly?
- Do you drink tea or coffee regularly?
- Do you exercise regularly?
- Do you follow a low-calorie diet?
- Are you recovering from an injury?
- Do you suffer from colds and/or flu regularly?
- Are you pregnant or breastfeeding?
- Do you actively or passively smoke? (Just so you know, the answer to this question is yes, we all passively smoke.)
- Do you live in or near a city?
- Do you drink tap water?
- Do you ever experience stress or anxiety?
- Are you exposed to toxins regularly?
- Do you suffer joint pain or conditions?
- Do you suffer from respiratory or skin issues?
- Do you have high cholesterol or blood pressure?
- Are you concerned about type II diabetes or other diseases?
- Are you on any medication, prescribed or over the counter?
- Are you interested in optimal well-being?

If you got through that list of questions without answering 'yes' to any of them, we need to talk – I want to know your secret! However, I'm assuming you registered at least one yes, certainly to the last question. Am I right? That being the case, if you are serious about changing things then I would recommend you start supplementing with a basic foundation of nutrients: multivitamin/minerals, anti-oxidants, omega-3, *Rhodiola* and probiotic as a starting point.

Now that we've identified we all need to supplement, the next question that needs to be answered is: which supplements do you choose? This is a cause of much confusion and scepticism. The statement that 'supplements are expensive urine' is correct for synthetically produced tablets, but not for organically grown plant-based supplements.

I'm not going to mention any specific brands. I am going to tell you what to look for and what to avoid and arm you with the questions to ask, so you can find the best product for you and your family. I think it would be fair to say you are looking for products as close as possible to nature. In other words, those that are made from real, raw plant material and are simply concentrated food matter.

Unfortunately, these products are hard to find, but they are a dozen times more effective than anything synthetic. In a general sense, there are effectively three types of nutritional supplements:

- *Compounds or oxides*: the most common form of supplement. Most of the brands you think of when you consider vitamins and minerals will generally fall into this category. They are cheaper to buy because they are synthetically produced by taking different nutritional compounds and artificially creating a tablet. The main problem with this type of supplement is that, because it's not naturally occurring, the body will immediately reject it in the same way it deals with all processed foods. Instead of absorbing most of the nutrients in the tablet, the body will work to eliminate them. In other words, they *are* expensive urine. The main issues with a compound or oxide is the minimal absorption of nutrients and the negative impact on the liver as the body tries to eliminate this synthetic substance.

- *Chelated*: as compound or oxide supplements have a very low nutrient absorption rate, in some cases an amino acid is added to force absorption of the compound into the body. These supplements are referred to as being chelated. This may seem like a good thing, but if you think about it, can you see the problem here? There is a reason why the body is only allowing a small amount of the compound to be absorbed – that is, to protect itself from synthetic substances. To force a synthetic compound into the body can only create problems, just as forcing a square peg into a round hole does.

- *Natural, organic and plant based*: clearly this is the type of supplement I'm going to recommend to you. Now, let's not dance around the truth: any and every supplement is processed to some extent. However, the closer it is to nature, the more of the nutrients will be assimilated into the body. The plants will be grown on certified organic farms. The processing of the tablets will be quick and simple, maintaining the nutritional integrity of the plant. The tablet will be concentrated whole plant-food material. The tablet will include many different phyto-nutrients that, for most products, are lost in the manufacturing process. The absorption of this type of supplement into the body as beneficial nutrients will be 80 to 90 per cent compared to 10 to 20 per cent for compounds or oxides.

For your own benefit, don't just blindly believe what is advertised or what is told to you by a shop assistant. Remember: anything you put into your body is going to have an impact on your long-term health, so don't compromise when it comes to supplements. If it's cheap, I promise you it will be the most expensive thing you've ever purchased and consumed! First, there will be minimal absorption, so you'll have to take many more pills to get the same potency, and second, there will be a negative impact on your well-being as a result of the synthetic products you are consuming on a daily basis.

When buying supplements, it's important to remember three key principles. It's not about the ingredients so much; it's about the source of the ingredients. It's not about their potency; it's about absorption. It's not about their cost; it's about quality and value.

Ask the right questions

With that in mind, there are some questions I recommend you ask to be one hundred per cent sure you are spending your money wisely and impacting your health positively. If the person you are asking can't answer the questions, find someone in the store or online who can. If there is no-one who can satisfactorily answer the questions, run, don't walk, in the opposite direction and find another option. Remember that it's your well-being at stake.

In her book *Secrets of Supplements: The good, the bad, the totally terrific*, Dr Gloria Askew poses 10 totally terrific questions you should ask before purchasing vitamins, mineral and herbal supplements:

1. Is your multi-supplement a plant-based product that includes vitamins, minerals and phyto-nutrients?
2. If the multi-supplement is plant based, is it derived from a variety of plants?
3. If the multi-supplement is plant based and is derived from a variety of plants, does the manufacturer own their own land and grow, harvest and concentrate their plants?
4. Does the vitamin C supplement contain the whole plant concentrate, including associated phyto-nutrients?
5. Are the plants used in the supplements, certified organic from the soil to the seed up?
6. Is the disintegration time of the tablet about 30 minutes or less?
7. Does the manufacturer voluntarily adhere to good manufacturing practices from seed to end product and to the Council for Responsible Nutrition for its fish oil products?
8. Does the manufacturer assay their entire line for heavy metals, micro-biological contaminants and pollutants and desirable nutrient compounds?
9. Does the manufacturer publish bio-assays that you can easily access?
10. Does the manufacturer publish an oxygen radical absorbance capacity score on its anti-oxidants that is based on a wide range of free radical groups?

'Yikes,' I hear you saying, 'is it really worth going to that much effort?' Only you can answer that question; only you can decide whether it's important enough. If you are going to invest in supplements you are planning to put in your body and those of your children, on a daily basis, wouldn't you want to know? They are going to either enhance the chances of optimal well-being or potentially break it down. The good news is, when you have found the product(s) that ticks all the boxes, you can stop looking and asking.

But wait, there are more questions I would encourage you to ask – this time regarding the omega-3 or fish oil supplements that are so critical. If you remember, I spoke about the importance of deep sea cold water fatty fish oil to increase the omega-3 ratio in cell membranes and enhance their ability to allow nutrients to nourish the cells. You may need to go back and re-read the section in Chapter 10 if you want a refresher.

Here are five fabulous questions to ask when shopping for a good quality fish oil supplement:

- Are the fish used in the product wild or farmed?
- If they are wild, are they smaller fish, which are lower on the food chain, such as sardines, anchovies and menhaden?
- Has the product been tested for heavy metals?
- Does the manufacturer voluntarily adhere to good manufacturing practices from the Council for Responsible Nutrition for its fish oil products?
- Is there an anti-oxidant (like vitamin E) in the capsule to prevent the possibility of oxidation?

I think I should explain the last question. Many oils, including fish oil, are sensitive to temperature. Once the oil is heated to a certain temperature the oil can begin to oxidise. In other words, it can become rancid, even carcinogenic. Adding vitamin E, a powerful anti-oxidant, prevents the threat of oxidation.

For vegans or vegetarians who don't eat fish and won't take fish oil, getting the most beneficial source of omega-3 fatty acids can be difficult. While there are plant-based sources of omega-3, they are far less usable by the cells and body. Alternative medicine proponent Dr Joseph Mercola says: 'While a tiny amount of the ALA [alpha-lipoic acid] you consume can be converted by your body into long-chain omega-3, it's a highly inefficient strategy and nowhere near as helpful as supplying "straight" DHA and EPA [both omega-3 fatty acids] from marine sources.'

So, for all you anti-fish consumers out there, get ready to consume a lot of flaxseeds, flaxseed oils, leafy greens, chia seeds and walnuts and any quality plant-based omega-3 supplement you can find. Again, with every supplement, the questions above should be satisfactorily answered before putting any type of product into your amazing and vulnerable body.

Swimming in a different gene pool

I want to finish this chapter as I started it: with an inspiring story about a friend of mine. Peter has an 'impressive' family history, as he describes it. His dad died at age 50 from a heart attack. His brother died at age 45 from a heart attack, after having a stroke at 40. His mother died after a stroke at age 71. He has two sisters and a brother who all have high blood pressure, high cholesterol and weight issues and have had double heart bypass surgery. All his siblings are taking medications. His aunt has a 60 per cent blockage in her carotid artery. His uncle has a 99 per cent blockage in his carotid artery. His grandparents all passed away with diabetes, high blood pressure and high cholesterol.

I don't know about you, but that's tiring and stressful for me to just read! Looking at his history, it would be pretty understandable to expect that Peter would very likely follow in similar footsteps. Well, this is why Peter is an incredibly inspiring person: he chose a different outcome for himself. He is currently 57 years of age and as fit, lean and healthy as a man many years younger. How could this be, considering the gene pool he was swimming in? Simple: he chose to get out of it and create and swim in a new gene pool.

His wife, a medical scientist, strongly encouraged him to make an appointment with a leading interventional cardiologist to find out where he was really at. When your wife strongly encourages, you listen. This doctor took one look at his family history and, without any further examination, immediately recommended Peter take aspirin to thin his blood and then stay on it for the rest of his life. Peter objected to any form of chemical with side effects, and he refused any procedure that would be invasive to his body. It took a lot of courage for Peter to not succumb to the fear strategy employed by his doctor. He was confident, however, that he had taken control of his own health and would not compromise it with synthetic and invasive options.

He finally agreed to a non-invasive angiography and would then consider other alternatives based on the results. Just as Peter had expected, the outcome of this test was positive and there was 'no evidence of any coronary heart disease'. As you can imagine, this astounded, intrigued and impressed the doctor, who advised Peter to keep doing whatever he was doing. Are you interested to know what that is?

I can tell you that it's nothing out of the ordinary and it's nothing that you can't do, starting today. Peter became heavily involved in a strong and positive association and started deliberately focusing on his life purpose. This gave him the vision, motivation, inspiration and impetus to take control of his life and his well-being and consequently he has made significant changes in his thinking, consumption, eating and exercise habits.

Peter committed to doing 10,000 steps per day as a base for his physical activity regime. While he does not describe himself as athletic, he recently took up jogging to support his wife. As a result, he 'inadvertently' ran the last seven kilometres of the 2016 Paris marathon as he was encouraging her in her first marathon! Peter introduced meditation into his life 20 years ago after his brother's death. This 20-minute ritual twice daily provides him a strong foundation of calm thinking and soulfulness.

Peter eats the way he knows he should be eating – the same way you know you should be eating. He uses waterless cookware and eats lots of fresh, natural and organic foods. He drinks only purified water and has a quality air purifier in his home. He is on a strict regime of organically grown food supplements including multivitamin/minerals, omega-3, anti-oxidants, *Rhodiola*, vitamins B and C and plant protein powder, just to name a few. He is leaving nothing to chance! There is no sign of any chemicals or medications in Peter's day; is it any wonder he has defied his genetic odds and is now swimming in a clear, fresh and healthy gene pool?

Putting the pieces in place

The nutritional piece is a large and sometimes overwhelming piece of the wellness puzzle. There are so many different books, resources and angles provided by a wide and varied range of people for all expanses of the wellness landscape. Even in this book, I've covered a lot of information, ideas and concepts over the last six chapters. I hope you're not feeling too confused, but instead feel empowered and excited that nature provides the nutrients you need and that all the amazing benefits that go with it are within your reach.

If I were to simplify and summarise here I would say:

- Eat breakfast within 10 to 15 minutes of getting out of bed and eat every 60 to 90 minutes throughout the day. This will help to keep the metabolic fire burning.
- Add quality protein to each meal or snack to help slow the release of sugar into the blood and help to sustain energy and further enhance metabolism.
- Look after your cells and allow them to do what they do so well by increasing omega-3 fatty acid intake and reducing your omega-6 and trans fat intake. In other words, eat less processed food and more fish and vegetables and don't be afraid of some saturated fat in moderation.
- Protect and increase your good gut bacteria by eating natural foods, fermented foods, prebiotics and a quality probiotic supplement.
- Purify your thinking and your environment to reduce the incidence of toxins, free radicals and cortisol.
- Pure water flushes toxins out of the body, so aim to drink one litre (34 fluid ounces) before eating each day. Consume lots of anti-oxidant–rich food to neutralise dangerous free radicals. *Rhodiola* regulates cortisol, so find a quality supplement and take them to start your day.

- Get a controlled amount of sun on your unprotected skin to make sure vitamin D is plentiful in your body.
- Choose certified organically grown foods wherever possible and get on a quality raw food plant-based supplement regime to make sure you have all the nutrients you require for optimal well-being.

Interestingly, many of the food choices you make will overlap and benefit you in many of the areas I've talked about in the previous chapters and summarised above. So start now – yes, I mean now. The minute you put down this book to go for a snack, why not get started? This second, make the choices that will put and keep you on the path to being lean and fabulous, energised and unstoppable and healthy and on purpose.

 Key questions and action steps

1. How much time do you spend in the sun on a weekly basis?
2. Could you prioritise the time to take yourself and your family out to get the recommended amount of vitamin D?
3. Are you consistently taking supplements for optimal well-being?
4. Based on what you know now, are they the best ones for you and your well-being?
5. Would you be willing to go and ask the right questions and get your hands on the products that will give you that amazing feeling of well-being you're looking for?
6. If you're overwhelmed, I'd be happy for you to contact me and ask me what I would recommend from a supplementation point of view. My email address is andrew@andrewjobling.com.au.

References/resources

https://www.myfooddata.com/articles/high-vitamin-D-foods.php

https://health.howstuffworks.com/wellness/food-nutrition/vitamin-supplements/how-much-vitamin-d-from-sun1.htm

https://sunwarrior.com/healthhub/natural-sunscreen-alternatives

https://articles.mercola.com/sites/articles/archive/2016/09/11/omega-3-from-plants-vs-marine-animals.aspx

Secrets of Supplements: The good, the bad, the totally terrific, Gloria Askew, Jerre Paquette & Carole Jeffries (eds), Phyte Media Inc., 2008

'Eat Your Suncreen', Bec Farah, *LivingNow*, Jan/Feb 2017, pages 48-51

The power of whole food
All food is good!

I truly believe all food is good; there are just some foods we should eat more of and some foods we should eat less of.

The last thing I need to do with this nutritional piece is talk about an empowering yet challenging subject, one that is often neglected, glossed over or swept under the carpet. If you are reading this book thinking that the author – me, that is – is some perfect robot that never eats anything other than fruits, vegetables, whole foods, natural proteins and healthy fats and drinks only purified water, you are wrong! I'm here to squash that theory right now. I love indulgence food as much as anyone else; I believe that indulgence foods are and should be a part of a healthy and enjoyable eating plan.

I love chocolate. I enjoy pizza. I am a sucker for ice-cream. I don't drink soft drink, but I do enjoy an alcoholic drink every now and then. So the exciting news for you is that I'm certainly not suggesting you give up all those foods. I just want you to understand where and how they fit into your weekly eating regime, and the mindset and decision-making process around choosing to consume them.

In society today, it's many of these indulgence foods that are blamed as the reason why so many people are overweight and unhealthy. It's almost like we are saying that as we are sleeping, ice-cream magically sneaks into the house, up the stairs and into our bedroom and forces its way into our mouths. Impossible, right? People all over the world are blaming the foods they eat for their health issues. Instead, maybe they should be blaming themselves for deliberately putting the food into their mouths, chewing it and swallowing it into their own bodies.

We are all living in an educated and information-rich world. There is no shortage of resources about which foods should be eaten more and which foods we should consume moderately. For anyone in a Western civilisation to say they were unaware of the health risks of any processed, synthetic or fast food that they choose to consume is a lie. This now includes you, if you honestly didn't know before right now. Whether you eat the food or not is totally up to you but, if you do, to then blame that food or to say you were unaware of the potential health risks is no longer an option. Make wise choices.

As I have already mentioned I, like anybody, love certain foods. I also believe eating some of the foods I have mentioned is an important part of my eating regime, because it provides wonderful enjoyment for me. That is healthy! The most important message I want to get across in this chapter is that it's not the food you consume that's the cause of any health issues, it's the reason why you are eating it that is the cause. This is where we will spend much of our time in this chapter.

I truly believe all food is good: there are just some foods we should eat more of and some foods we should eat less of. The worst thing you, or anyone, can do is label any food as 'bad'. Why? Because the second you label a food as bad and then eat it, what does that say about you? If you eat bad food, you must be bad. If you make unhealthy food choices, doesn't that make you unhealthy? If you put junk food in your mouth, wouldn't that make you a junk yard? If you have a 'cheat' day, doesn't that make you a cheat? I mean, let's face it: is chocolate bad? No way, it's fantastic. Is ice-cream unhealthy? Not to me it isn't. Is pizza junk food? Not to the Italians it isn't.

From now on I want you to consider all food as great. You now know that there are some foods you should eat more of and some foods less, right? As I already mentioned, the reason for eating the indulgence foods is the main issue. The food itself is just sitting there to be eaten, but it will never force its way into your mouth – you will do that. If you find you are over-indulging on these foods, then you need to explore your reasons for it. I will help you with that shortly. First, let's think of all the foods we love to eat but keep getting told are unhealthy, junk, bad and rubbish.

Let's go wild. There are times I eat ice-cream and love it, chocolate and won't give it up, pizza and can taste it now, Chinese yum cha and love those dumplings, cake (sometimes two slices) and many other yummy foods. What about you? How about burgers, fried chicken, chips and fries, dim sims, lollies, soft drinks, Coco Pops, Froot Loops, fish 'n' chips, biscuits, pastries and many other mouth-watering delicacies? They are all great, right? As long as we make a sensible decision about eating them.

What do I mean by sensible decision to eat them? I mean a decision not driven by a craving, an emotional response or a feeling of low self-worth. I will get into these things in more detail soon. If your decision to eat an indulgence food is made with control, knowing that a moderate amount is enough (and deep down, you know what a moderate amount is) and then you will get back to eating the foods that are on the 'eat more of' list, I say go for it and enjoy it. This is a sensible approach to indulgence, not one driven by a strong and possibly dangerous emotional response.

I'm not a psychologist, but I have seen all of the things I'm about to touch on many times over. If you recognise anything I'm talking about as a behaviour you regularly adopt, could I suggest you reach out to someone you trust for help? It may not seem like a big deal right now, but it could turn into something that controls and harms you in the long term.

Cravings

Despite what you may think, cravings are not normal, not good for you, and are not going to lead to a happy and healthy life. I talk to many people who tell me they are a chocoholic, like it's some type of medical condition. It's not a medical condition; it's the body craving energy. People tell me they can't survive without sugar, caffeine, pizza, soft drinks, energy drinks, bread and many other foods that we should place on the 'eat less of' list. People tell me they can't stop at eating just a small meal and have issues with portion control. Again, they talk as if it's some type of chemical imbalance or physical affliction, when it's simply the body craving the right food and more energy.

What a craving does is give immediate feedback that we are not giving our body what it needs. The mistake many people make is to react to their cravings, which keeps the craving happening, rather than responding and removing the cause of the craving. A couple of things to understand about cravings are they are things we bring on ourselves, there is no quick-fix solution, and you can't beat a craving with willpower. Let's look at a typical scenario that impacts many lives, and then let's look at a way to remove the problem forever.

John is an ambitious young man trying to prove himself in the law firm by which he has just been employed. In addition to his new demanding job, he plays a high level of competitive basketball, requiring three or four training sessions and games after work and on weekends each week. When he gets home from his hectic day, he does some research, watches some TV, connects with friends on social media and finally falls into bed exhausted. Despite being active, happy and hard working, John is starting to struggle with his work, sporting and social commitments. Consequently, his work standard is dropping, his sporting performance is not as good as it used to be, his energy is lacking, he is surprisingly putting on weight and he is starting to get a little unusually moody.

If we look at John's eating regime, it's actually pretty easy to see why all these things are happening. Being so tired when he goes to bed, he finds it hard to get up the next day. He hits snooze on his alarm several times before he is able to drag himself out of bed. When he does finally get up he is running late, so he has no time to sit down for a good breakfast. Instead, he grabs a processed muesli bar if anything and a cup of coffee. His partner has done the right thing for him and packed fruit, vegetables, nuts, a protein bar and a nutrient-rich salad and meat multigrain sandwich for him.

John has so many things on at work he simply forgets to eat a snack in the morning, and in fact the idea of fruit and vegetable sticks is pretty unappealing to him. Because his body is now running on empty, it's calling out for energy and he is starting to crave sugar. He struggles through the morning, wondering why he is having trouble concentrating. At lunchtime, with such a strong craving for sugar, processed foods and a quick fix, he ignores the beautifully fresh and natural lunch his partner has prepared and goes to the local cafe to buy chips, pies, dim sims, chocolate and another coffee. As he is devouring this food he knows deep down he should be eating the fruit, vegetables and beautiful sandwich his partner prepared, but he can't help himself. It's like someone or something else is controlling his body.

The result of his dumping of sugar and processed food into his body has an immediate and dramatic effect on his blood sugar levels. They rise quickly, his energy levels fly, and for a short time he feels great. However, what goes up must come down. John's pancreas produces insulin to get his blood sugar levels down quickly to protect his health. The impact of his blood sugar levels falling is that within a short time he feels more tired and lethargic and has stronger cravings than before. He heads into meetings after lunch with a seriously affected ability to focus and his behaviour starts to change. He is becoming moody and intolerant and starts to cause some conflict in the office, leading to reprimands and punishment from the partners.

After work John heads to basketball training. He can't understand why his performance and stamina are declining, and why when he was once so good at the sport he is now struggling to keep a spot in the team. At night he comes home exhausted and ravenous. He over-eats many of the foods that are sitting on the 'eat less of' list. He can't seem to help it; he is craving so badly and just wants to feel better. Sugar seems to be the only solution. He can't focus on his work and so falls asleep in front of the TV and then goes to bed exhausted, fatigued and full.

The next day John wakes up and struggles to get out of bed, and the whole negative cycle continues. Can you see how cravings have totally controlled and devastated John's life, activities and aspirations? As I mentioned, cravings are not a medical condition, but they will control your life and well-being. Getting rid of them is simple: by doing exactly what I discussed in the previous chapters.

In John's case, because he wanted to change things, he decided to get out of bed when his alarm went off, even though he didn't feel like. He then had the time to sit down and eat a great, natural and energy-giving breakfast. He set up a reminder system on his phone to notify him when it was time to eat again. This time, he stuck to eating the beautiful food his partner had packed for him. No more cravings, no more spending money at the cafe, no more lethargy and no more Mr Cranky-pants! John was back to his best: doing well at work, on his basketball team and in all the other areas of life. He is lean, fit and feeling fabulous, all because he sorted out his cravings.

Moods

The question is: do our moods control our eating, or does our eating control our moods? This is an interesting one to ponder, and I would say the answer is … yes! Yes, our eating can control our moods, and our moods can control our eating. Either one can get a crazy cycle started, and then both can keep it spinning. What do I mean by a crazy cycle?

Once on this cycle, it's very difficult to get off it. In the example I discussed with John, he was well and truly on the crazy cycle and it was significantly impacting his life and his well-being. He had to make a serious, deliberate and uncomfortable decision to get off it. I will discuss emotional eating more in the next section, but for now let's talk about how to control one part of the crazy cycle that will stop it in its tracks. That is, your moods.

The biggest misconception many people have is that they are not in control of their moods. We too often believe moods are dictated by our circumstances.

The crazy cycle

Bad mood: from external situation; angry, sad, anxious and so on. **Comfort food**: soft drink, chocolate, processed foods and so on.

Uncontrolled eating: due to craving soft drinks, chocolate, processed foods and so on. **Mood swings**: blood sugar levels rise and then fall, leading to lethargy, cravings and bad moods.

The crazy cycle.

What I mean by this is, if things are going well for us then we are in a good mood. If things are not going as we would like, then we are in a bad mood. I hear it all the time, and in fact I've said it myself: 'It's not my fault, I was angry because so and so said/did this to me.' It may be easy for you to say, 'I'm in a bad mood because I didn't get the result I wanted in that test/project.'

What I need you to understand clearly – and this will revolutionise your well-being and your life – is that you control your moods. If you remember, I have already discussed that our thoughts control our emotional state, and our emotional state is effectively our mood. You and I get to choose our thoughts, therefore, we control our moods. If we control our moods, we can get ourselves off the crazy cycle whenever we want.

When someone does or says something to you that you don't like, you can choose your thoughts about this. Instead of thinking: 'It's not fair', 'I don't like that person', 'I will get them back', 'What's wrong with me?' or any other negative

The energising cycle

Good mood: choosing to see the best and be grateful.

Good food choices: wanting to eat well and stay healthy.

In control of eating: due to feeling great and wanting to be better. High-quality foods consumed.

Feeling great: good energy, being happy with a positive and optimistic focus.

The energising cycle.

type of thought, why not try something different? Instead, you could choose to think: 'That's okay, they are entitled to their opinion', 'I am now determined to prove them wrong', 'I can learn from this and get better', 'I feel sorry for that person; they must be going through a bad time to say/do that to me'.

When you don't get the job or other result you wanted, you might be thinking: 'I'm not smart', 'I'll never be good enough to get the promotion I want', 'Why can others do it, and I can't?', 'I'm useless'. Instead, you could try thinking: 'Okay, that was not so good, but I can improve', 'I will learn from this and be better next time', 'This is great because now I get a chance to improve'.

When you choose a positive thought in response to an undesirable situation, your mood will be more positive and therefore the action you take will be positively impacted. As we are talking about the crazy eating cycle here, the choice you will make around eating will get you straight off this crazy cycle. If you control your thoughts, and therefore your moods, you will automatically make better food choices and you are off the crazy cycle and onto the energising cycle.

As you can see, the energising cycle is the best place to be as it will keep you feeling fabulous and making great food choices and therefore help attain and maintain optimal well-being. The most important thing you need to know is that you are in control of your moods because you choose your thoughts. Choose good ones!

Emotional eating

I have covered a lot of this area in the previous two sections. As I mentioned, if you can make better choices to help remove cravings, you will have more level energy and therefore be in a better situation to control any emotional situations that may arise. When you realise you get to choose the thoughts that control your moods, this will also help you stay on top of making better decisions based on undesirable situations. Now, having said all of that, as humans we are all affected by negative emotions in our life, and as much as we may have control over our thoughts, there are times when we are all angry, sad, resentful, bitter, fearful and anxious.

That being the case, if binge eating or starving yourself is your response to any of these emotional situations, then you should think about some alternate responses. Certain foods may give short-term comfort when we are emotional. Foods such as chocolate, ice-cream, lollies, cakes, pizzas, chips and many other indulgence foods seem to be where we go for comfort. Again, these are not bad foods; they are just foods we should eat less of and certainly not foods we should eat based on a strong emotional response. Alternatively, starving themselves may be the chosen response for some people. If we allow ourselves to be controlled by our emotions and simply excuse poor choices because of our emotional state, then we totally lose control of our well-being and our life.

When you and I are under stress, food can be a great relief. When the pressure of performance is on, food can be a possible short-term distraction from the reality of what needs to be done and the stress and fear of poor results.

When you get a result that is not the one you want and you are angry or upset, food can offer short-term comfort. When you are having trouble getting on with certain people and there is some conflict or even bullying, food is always there and can provide reassurance in those times when you need it. When you feel inadequate, not able to deal with demands or not happy with your performance at work or in a team, it can be food you turn to to help relieve some of the pain. The only issue with using food as your comfort or your escape is that it will never solve the problem. It only ever offers short-term solace, and will cause many more problems in the future.

Emotional eating is simply a pattern we create for ourselves. Maybe as a child, when you were unhappy, sad or upset your parents gave you food as a pacifier. You learned from a young age that when you feel any of these emotions food is the place to go, but it doesn't have to be. You can change the pattern and you are in control of your response. There are many better options when you feel that trigger or pull towards food.

The first thing is to be able to recognise any moments that would normally trigger you to head for the pantry or fridge. The instant you feel the negative emotion – and if you can identify it before you put those chocolate biscuits in your mouth – you can change the action you would normally take, which in this case is eating. If you change your response you can change your results, and there are some great ideas as alternatives in that moment you would normally feel drawn to food.

At a demanding time in life when you are stressed, some form of exercise is a great way to relieve the stress and clear the head. Go for a walk or run, hit a boxing bag, kick a football or do a short period of some physical activity. When you get a result that you are not happy with, immediately talk to someone who can give you a proper perspective about it, such as your partner, your parents, a mentor or a trusted and supportive friend. When you are having trouble with conflict or bullying, immediately go to work on your self-image. Tell yourself you are a good person, think about your own great qualities, understand the other person is having some personal issues (which is why they are being mean to you), talk to someone who loves you and, finally, eat some good-quality food and do some exercise. You will feel great after all of these things. Whenever you feel inadequate or not good enough, immediately think about your strengths and write them down, and get excited about the fact that you can always learn, improve and try again.

Any of these strategies, and any others you can think of, can easily replace the emotional eating you are doing. Just remember to catch yourself before taking that first bite, and ask yourself what a better response to the way you're feeling would be. It won't be easy to start with, but with practice you will soon be able to effortlessly deal with the demands and challenges of life in a positive and optimally healthy way.

Eating disorders

To repeat, I'm not a psychologist, but I have seen and dealt with many people with eating disorders, even people very close to me. All I want to really say to you is, if you feel like your eating is covering up something, is a way to run from something, is protecting you from something or if the choices you are making are to help with your self-esteem or your body image, please go and talk to someone who can give you some perspective. What starts off as a seemingly logical and harmless decision can easily spiral into a dangerous and even life-threatening condition.

Zoe was a 13-year-old girl who had just started at a new school. She was an only child with professional parents who were always too busy working to really spend quality time with her. From a young age she started to develop feelings of inadequacy and that she was not really unconditionally loved by her parents, as they would always put work before her. Through feelings of guilt, her parents tried to spoil her in material ways. They always bought her new clothes, toys and gifts and allowed her to do things that were perhaps not the best for her health.

Zoe started emotionally eating chocolate, biscuits and cake to comfort and protect herself from these feelings of rejection. I'm sure you know the result of this type of eating? Yes, she started to put on weight, and while not obese she was becoming a little plumper every day. To compound her issues her father was often relocated with his job and Zoe was moved from school to school, never really being able to settle into one school. She started experiencing teasing and bullying because she was always the new girl and because her weight was steadily increasing. After every miserable day at her new school she would come home, lock herself in her room and binge on chocolate to cover up her immediate pain and rejection. The problem was that with each mouthful of chocolate she started loathing herself a little more, to the point where she really didn't see any value or worth in herself at all.

After moving to yet another school and suffering all sorts of bullying and name calling, Zoe decided enough was enough. It was time to take control and change her life, so she made the decision to lose weight, look fabulous and try to get back some self-esteem. She started on a regime of rigorous exercise and started to eat much less than she was used to. As she started losing weight, although she did begin to feel better about herself, she still didn't like what she saw in the mirror. Every time she looked at herself she could hear the comments she was so used to hearing ringing in her ears: 'Hey, fatty!', 'Here comes tubby', 'Watch out, she might sit on you', 'Be careful you don't break the chair' and many more.

Although she was starting to look better, Zoe couldn't see it. She still felt fat and unattractive, so she began to eat less and less. When she had to eat in front of people she would, but then she would go and make herself vomit to get rid of the calories. She would dispose of the beautiful lunch her mother had packed for her and pretend she had eaten it. She was spiralling into a very bad place. As she lost more and more weight, it was obvious to everyone except herself that she had a serious eating disorder. In her mind and eyes she was still overweight and ugly.

This eating disorder ran for many years, into her early 20s. Over that time it impacted her energy levels, her moods, her relationships and her study and work, and there were even several occasions Zoe found herself in hospital and fighting for her life. Finally, she realised she had a problem and that enough was enough. She allowed her parents to help her and, eventually, with the right counsel and support, she started to build back her self-esteem, accept herself and start on a healthy and energy-giving eating plan. She is a happy and healthy young lady today.

Zoe's problem was not food; anyone who has some type of eating disorder doesn't have a food or eating problem. What they have is a self-image and self-love, or more appropriately self-loathing, problem. This a serious emotional issue that can't be solved simply with an eating plan. It needs love, support and helping the person feel loved and accepted no matter what they look like. Again, I want to stress, if you feel like you are heading down this path please reach out for help. There are many people who love and accept you, but the only person who needs to love and accept you is you.

Learning to love food

We have to eat, right? As you now know, we really need to eat great food multiple times every day to be lean, fit, energised, healthy, happy and be able to achieve the amazing things in life that are important to us. So, if the truth is that we need to eat, what a tragedy if eating is a stressful and unenjoyable activity. I want to help you love food, love eating and love the benefits you get from it.

Let's look at the three main benefits of eating:

- enjoyment
- energy
- optimal well-being

You will notice I didn't put weight loss. Why? Because weight loss, or more accurately fat loss will happen as a natural consequence of these three things. It is my desire you will get to the point where you love eating, won't be afraid of certain foods and won't binge for the wrong reasons, but instead create a wonderfully enjoyable, energising and wellness-inducing eating regime that you can maintain forever.

Enjoyment

My theory is this: if it's not enjoyable it won't last. Enjoying your eating means that you not only eat the indulgence foods you like in moderation, but you learn to love eating fruits, vegetables, great proteins and healthy fats, because they help you achieve your goals this year, next year and on into your life.

I'm not sure if you are anything like I used to be: I loved eating meat and proteins; I didn't mind eating rice, pasta and bread; but I could do without eating fruits and vegetables. I just didn't enjoy them as much as other foods. As a child and teen, I was a real pain in the backside when it came to eating. I was fussy, I was picky and I was stubborn. My mother tried many things to get me to eat vegetables. She would mix them in with mashed potato. She would hide them in pies, pasties and other baked foods. She would cover them in melted cheese. She would wrap them up in meat. She was very persistent and very creative but, alas for her, I was too clever. I would find them, pick them out and leave them on the side of the plate.

She then tried to explain to me why eating fruits and vegetables was important. She told me health regulations reported I was meant to eat five to eight serves of fruits and vegetable every day. I didn't care. She told me they were good for my health. I took no notice. She withheld desserts and treats until I ate them. I always convinced her to give me the desserts and treats anyway. I was a total brat, and I'm surprised she never resorted to physical means. I would have slapped myself!

Then one day my mother stopped trying to convince me to eat fruits and vegetables. One day she stopped persisting, stopped trying to hide them, stopped trying to make me do something I clearly was not going to do. She was, as are all mothers, far more switched on than I ever gave her credit for. You see, this withdrawal of nagging me to eat fruits and vegetables coincided with my declaration that I was going to become a professional footballer.

My mother was a very smart lady. She worked in the library at a school and found some articles about, and interviews with, professional footballers, sports nutritionists and coaches. These articles and interviews all talked about the importance of good nutrition, and why eating lots of fruits and vegetables was critical for elite athletes. She just happened to leave these documents lying around where I could see them. One day my curiosity got the better of me, and I started to read them.

That night at dinner, Mum put my meal in front of me. On the plate was a beautifully cooked steak and a pile of mashed potatoes. There weren't any other vegetables on the plate at all. I looked at the plate, I looked back at Mum, I looked at the plate again and I said, 'Hey, Mum, can I have some other vegetables please?' She went and got me a pile of peas, carrots, broccoli and cauliflower. I ate all of it and enjoyed it, and have not stopped eating vegetables ever since!

How did she do it? How did she turn me around? How did she get me to become an avid and obsessed fruit and vegetable eater, when she could never previously get me to eat even the smallest amount? What was her special secret? My mother realised she couldn't tell me what to do. It was just painful for me and frustrating for her. She worked out that eating better had to be my decision, not hers. She realised the only way I would ever decide to eat more fruits and vegetables, and enjoy it, was if it somehow helped me achieve the things that were important to me. At that time in my life I was an obsessed young man; my eyes were football shaped. It's all I thought about, talked about and cared about. My very clever mother realised that if I could see a connection between eating more nutritious foods and success as a professional footballer, then no longer would eating vegetables be a painful chore but instead an exciting opportunity to be a better and more successful footballer.

It worked like a dream. Those same vegetables I resisted and gagged on for so long I now gobbled down with ease. Every time I chewed and swallowed the nutrient-rich food I could feel it making me healthier, more energised and a more equipped athlete. It had nothing to do with the fruits and vegetables and everything to do with what they were doing to me and for me. I have been a passionate fruit and vegetable eater ever since, and it's absolutely helped me in every area of my life to date and will continue to do so as I work towards living beyond 100 years old.

Now, every day, I love food. I enjoy a great breakfast because it fuels me for the day. I look forward to snacking every hour or so as it keeps me more energised, focused and productive. I can't wait for lunch and dinner, because with every bite I can feel the food nourishing my body and keeping me strong, lean and healthy. I love every opportunity to eat some indulgence foods such as ice-cream, pizza, chocolate and yummy drinks. I would encourage you to eat a variety of wonderful foods and enjoy it, because you can't live, function or thrive without it. Enjoy fresh natural foods most of the time, and in moderation eat some of those indulgence foods you love. Just make sure the reasons why you are eating them are the right reasons. You know what I mean, don't you?

Energy

Energy is what makes us go. Fuel in the car is the only way it will move. Electricity is the only way we can get light and power. Gas is how we end up with a hot shower. Food is the fuel for your body, to get and keep it moving so you can do all the things you want and need to do. I want to encourage you, the majority of the time, to choose the foods that will give you optimal energy.

This analogy makes the point beautifully. You may or may not be into horses, but let's say you owned a racehorse. That racehorse will cost a lot of money and take a lot of money to maintain; I know this from bitter personal experience. The only way to get money back and make a profit is if the horse wins races. Then you can collect your winnings and the prize money. Now, if the only way of making money is if the horse wins races, it needs to run faster than the other horses, right? If you had the choice of feeding the horse Froot Loops, chocolate, fried chips and soft drink or high-quality and nutrient-rich natural foods, which would you choose? It sounds like a dumb question, doesn't it? Of course you would choose the best food to maximise energy and the chances of the horse winning races.

That being the case, are you more important than a racehorse? The answer is yes. What will maximise the chances of you having optimal energy, feeling great, performing better and achieving more? Will it be Froot Loops, chocolate, fried chips and soft drink or high-quality and nutrient-rich natural foods? You know the answer, so can I encourage you again to start doing it more?

Optimal well-being

It may be hard to think about this if you are already full of energy and feeling like you are healthy. There is, however, no better feeling than optimal well-being. It's the combination of all the things I have already spoken about, and the things I will discuss in the next chapters. My goodness, the life you can live and the things you can do when your health is fantastic! On the flipside, the things you will miss and be unable to do due to poor health are not even worth thinking about, and something if you follow the ideas in this book you will never have to experience.

I want to encourage you to think only about optimal well-being; it really is the only option. Having an exciting vision, having faith that everything will work out, thinking positively and being very aware about everything that goes into your body will enable a life you probably right now can't even imagine. I did not ever imagine the life I live today when I was young. As I sit here and write my ninth book, I have to pinch myself and wonder how I got here. It happened because I never accepted average. It happened because I never accepted mediocre. It happened because I never allowed myself to be distracted or affected by the opinions of other people. It happened because I have, from an early age, always focused on my health and well-being. I am so very grateful to have made the choices I made, to be living the life I live today.

To have focus, energy, strength and a body that is functioning at a high level is the ticket to any success imaginable. This is all possible when you put the best fuel in your body that you can.

Putting the pieces in place

As I wrap up this chapter and the previous chapters on puzzle piece five of the wellness puzzle – nutrition – I want you to really think about the foods you eat and the reasons why you eat them. It is the **reasons why you eat** what and when you eat that is determining your future health, happiness and success, not **the food you are actually eating**. When you can identify the thoughts leading to the emotions that are influencing your choices, you can start to make the changes in thinking that will significantly change your actions, habits and therefore results.

All food is great, so you can enjoy your indulgence foods without guilt. The condition is that eating them is NOT a craving, an emotional response or a way to mask feelings or deal with self-image issues. When you choose foods because you enjoy them but can exercise control and moderation then get back to wonderfully natural and nutrient-rich foods, you are well on the way to optimal well-being.

 Key questions and action steps

1. Think about your relationship with food. Do you really enjoy eating, or does is create stress in your life? Is it a crutch, a cover or a response to certain feelings you experience, or is it a wonderful experience and you feel good after every time you eat? These questions are important ones to consider.

2. Would you say you were mostly on the crazy cycle or the energising cycle? If you are finding yourself on the crazy cycle much of the time, what are some things you can change to get yourself off it and onto the energising cycle?

3. In what situations, if any, do you find yourself resorting to emotional eating? What are some alternative things you could do instead of eating?

4. Honestly, can you see yourself or someone you know with signs that may be leading to an eating disorder of any type? If so, would you be willing to ask for help for yourself or advice as to how you can help the person you are concerned about?

5. The key reasons why we eat are enjoyment, energy and optimal well-being. Think about how you get enjoyment out of food. Think about how you can change your eating to ensure you have more energy to do the things you want. Think about how you can ensure you gain optimal well-being through your eating plan, and what changes you can make.

6

Have faith in what you cannot see

For just a short time, give up the need for being in control, for validation from external sources and for thinking luck has anything to do with outcomes in your life. Feel the peace that comes from having faith that everything is going to be okay.

I'm going to get right out of my comfort zone here. I'm going to write some stuff that you may like or not like, agree with or disagree with, that may make you feel comfortable or uncomfortable. For that I make no apologies. Even deciding to add this piece to the puzzle was a last-minute decision, made because of a gut feeling I had that something intangible was missing.

I want to make it very clear right from the beginning that, while I have a Christian belief, I'm not promoting any specific type of faith platform, belief system or religious affiliation in this chapter. What I'm suggesting is that, unless we have some type of faith in a higher purpose, a guiding light, spiritual enlightenment, the universe or even just the belief that everything happens for a reason, then the world is a confusing, stressful and meaningless place.

I was raised in a loving family by parents I adore and for whom I am incredibly grateful. I had little to no exposure to any type of religious belief or spiritual affiliation. I was taught that if you work hard, do the right things and treat people right, everything will be okay. Now, while I still believe all of those qualities are important, I now understand there is more to it than that. We all need to have a faith if optimal well-being is our goal. You'll need to bear with me throughout this chapter, as I will do my best to unpack this powerful subject. In fact, you will need to have faith!

Let me throw a few definitions and interpretations of the word 'faith' at you.

The *Oxford Dictionary* has two definitions of 'faith':

1. Complete trust or confidence in someone or something.
2. Strong belief in the doctrines of a religion, based on spiritual conviction rather than proof.

Gospel singer Karen Wheaton says: 'Faith is believing that the things you cannot see are more real than the things you can see.'

In the Bible, Hebrews 11:1 states: 'Faith is the substance of things hoped for, the evidence of things not seen.'

An anonymous source puts it this way: 'Faith is seeing the light with your heart when all your eyes see is darkness.'

This from Martin Luther King Jr: 'Faith is taking the first step even when you don't see the whole staircase.'

Saint Augustine said: 'Faith is to believe what you do not see; the reward of this faith is to see what you believe.'

Author Philip Yancey's interpretation is: 'Faith is believing in advance what only makes sense in reverse.'

Faith is an inner knowing, confidence and peace that gives us perspective and, by its definition, removes stress and worry about external circumstances. Faith connects us to something bigger and more powerful than ourselves and provides comfort, certainty and peace of mind. It's interesting how faith and life works. When you believe and have faith in what you can't see, the answers, information, perspective and opportunities you want – or don't even know you want – seem to magically appear. Whether it's faith of a religious kind or whether it's a connectedness to the universe and a trust in its laws, faith is a powerful belief to own.

When we lose faith, we lose that connection to a higher source. That source may be a religion, a belief system, a spiritual path, a higher purpose or our wonderful universe. I was recently discussing this with a friend of mine who is now an intuitive healer. She told me she had been through the hapless, helpless and hopeless feeling of having no connection to a greater purpose. It was that time in her life when she spiralled into depression. She spoke about her turning point, when she decided enough was enough. Over time, with some introspection, she reconnected with her higher purpose and the depression was replaced with optimism. She now works with many people suffering depression to help them reconnect with their personal faith. She said the one thing each depressed person she works with has in common is this disconnection with faith of some kind.

I have another good friend, John, who is a pastor and is doing amazing work in his church and the community at large. Before I became Christian, John and I were talking, and at one point he stopped, looked at me and said: 'I feel like I need to discuss something with you.' He looked serious, like he had an important message for me. I responded a little nervously: 'Okay, John, what would you like to discuss?'

I know I'm not going to explain this as well as he did, but I'll do my best. He asked me about my beliefs and my purpose. I told him my purpose is to help people and to inspire them to get more out of themselves and their lives. He then asked me a question I had to really think about: *'What is your faith and what keeps you grounded?'* I thought about it, answered it somewhat superficially and immediately realised I had got it wrong.

John pulled out a piece of paper and drew a line down the middle. On one side he wrote the word 'external' and on the other side the word 'internal'. He went on to explain that most of the things that I had mentioned when he asked about what kept me grounded were external things: my work, my writing and even my marriage. By 'external' he meant they were things outside of me and my absolute control. He was trying to tell me that to rely on these things for peace and happiness was a risk, because at any time they could change. I hope you understand what I'm saying in this untidy way.

John went on to talk about 'internal' things; he was referring to faith. In his life, faith was fuelled by God and the Bible. He had an impenetrable faith that his path on earth was divinely led. I thought about it a bit more, and while at that time I was not a disbeliever, I had no strong religious affiliation. I thought about my faith in the universe. I told John I believe everything happens for a reason and that the universe provides me with what I need when I need it, to have, be and live the life I was destined to live. I think he was satisfied with my answer!

While the conversation with John was quite an uncomfortable one to have, I'm very grateful for it because it really highlighted to me the importance of a faith – in whatever shape it may take – if being optimally healthy is an aspiration of yours. Knowing with confidence that everything happens for a reason is a comforting thought, isn't it? To know that the people you meet, the confrontations you may face, the doors that will open and the lessons there to be learned will lead you to a better place takes the worry and stress out of your life. What are the biggest causes of dis-ease on the planet? Yes: worry, anxiety and stress.

I certainly haven't always believed in Christianity or faith in any way, shape or form. For much of my early life I was more interested in external validation to provide me with the feeling that I was a good, successful and popular person. I often speak about my professional football career. One of the main driving reasons for why I wanted to be a successful athlete was a need to be noticed, gain attention and be popular. It may sound shallow to you – as it now does to me – but it was where I was at the time.

I'm sure you can see the major problem associated with this superficial need. What do you think happened to my self-esteem, self-image and ego when I was sacked from the club at the tender age of 24? Not only was I no longer a professional sportsman, I was a rejected one. It had a seriously negative impact on my well-being and my life, and I took zero responsibility for it. I blamed everyone I could except the one person at fault – myself. I started justifying all my challenging circumstances, rather than take control. I threw the tantrum of all tantrums, instead of finding solutions. I held on to bitterness and resentment for many years.

Let's just analyse the outcome of my attitude and reaction to this event. First, as a result of my immature victim thinking and blaming, which I held on to for many years, I lost any opportunity to continue to play football at the highest level – I sabotaged my own career. Second, we've spoken in depth already about the impact of stress, anxiety, resentment and bitterness on a healthy body, so I inadvertently compromised my health and well-being. Third, I incorrectly connected my value as a human and happiness to that ego-driven image of a cool sportsman and I allowed it to erode my self-worth.

Then I moved into the fitness industry, which led me down an equally dangerous path and I became very body focused. This time, the personal recognition of my value came from my external body shape and the admiration of others. I trained too hard too often. I ate obsessively all of the time. While I got my body to an amazing state, I had to work hard, was continually stressed and sacrificed on a daily basis to maintain this unrealistic image. I look at myself back then and realise how high maintenance I was.

I needed constant validation from people to feed my fragile ego and self-esteem. If I wasn't performing to my peak every single time I would berate myself terribly and then rely on others to lift me back up. I was the most annoying person in the world to go out to dinner with. I would be very selective, choosing restaurants based on the menu to find meals I would eat. I would continually ask for meals to be changed and modified to suit my extreme tastes. It was not fun for me or the people I was dining with. It was stressful.

I'm not going to tell you any more embarrassing stories; you now know too much about me and my imperfections already! What I will say – as I look back over my life to where I am today – I've landed in an incredible place and one I wouldn't change for anything. How did it happen? It's hard to comprehend, especially when I think about all of the spontaneous decisions, poor choices and seemingly devastating circumstances that have littered my path to this point.

Here I am today, despite the fact that over my life I've dealt with numerous fears and insecurities, sustaining multiple brutal injuries as a footballer, the humiliation of being sacked on a public forum, recovering from many broken relationships, having failed in business, losing hundreds of thousands of dollars, working long hours and myself into the ground for many years, the heartbreak of losing my mother to cancer and countless other silly, embarrassing and dumb decisions! Despite all that, here I am: married to a lady I adore, following my passion and purpose, looking and feeling amazing and on track to live a long, happy and abundant life with no regrets.

If I'd known then what I know now I would just have had faith that everything that seemed undesirable at the time was exactly what I needed, and was leading me to where I am today. I wouldn't have been so fearful or insecure; I would've been calm and assured. I wouldn't have been humiliated by getting sacked; I would've been grateful. I wouldn't have been so stressed about work, businesses and money; I would've been excited it was teaching me the lessons I needed to learn. I wouldn't have been so devastated and crippled by the death of my mother; I would've been more joy filled that I knew her and proud to be able to share her legacy. I would never have been so heartbroken by getting dumped by many girls; I would've been thrilled that they would lead me to meeting my beautiful wife Laura. I wouldn't have worried about and dwelled on my poor choices so much; I would have learned the lessons, gained the perspective and moved on. I would have had faith!

I truly believe I've been led to this place. I believe that every decision I've made and every situation I've faced has moved me in a direction I didn't even consciously know at the time I wanted to head. I now totally trust that God and the universe deliver. At this time, I have absolute certainty that there are no accidents in life and that we create our own luck. I'm committed to the belief that things don't happen to us; they happen for us. I currently have unwavering faith that I am on track to create the amazing destiny that is available for me.

Here is something I previously wrote: 'The things in your life that seem bad at the time will open doors you didn't even consider, save you from the things you will be eternally grateful for, lead you to meet people you didn't know you wanted to meet and teach you things you had no idea you needed to or wanted to learn. Once you can think this way, believe that everything is good and trust that you are on the right path the sooner you will kick on in life.'

My point is this: I didn't need to worry, stress, fuss or fear as I was being led universally, divinely or whatever you want to call it – as are you. Can you see why having faith, belief and trust in a higher power than yourself is such an important quality to develop? Do you now understand how it can lead you to true happiness, amazing fulfilment and optimal well-being?

Depending on your beliefs, your attitudes and your openness to accept what I'm talking about in this chapter, you will know that inside of you and/ or on a spiritual level there is a guiding system that will always lead you in the right direction if you simply choose to have faith. If you are religious you will know exactly what I mean. If you trust in the universe and the law of attraction you will also know what I mean.

I'm now actually talking to the sceptics, the doubters and/or those who want so hard to believe and have faith, but to whom it sounds all too woo-woo or too good to be true. I can relate to you, because that was me.

Have faith in the laws of the universe

I think we can all agree that if you went to the top of a very tall building, out on the roof and over to the edge and then took another step, what would happen next is predictable. You don't need to understand the law of gravity

– you don't even have to agree with it – but on the way down you will know without a shadow of doubt that the law of gravity is truth.

What about the law of addition? Are you with me when I say that two plus two equals four? You don't need to think about it, hypothesise over it or debate it. No matter how you try it, two plus two always equals four. It is truth. Many years ago it wasn't truth; it started as someone's crazy idea. A caveman picked up two coconuts and then another two coconuts and asked (in caveman grunts), 'If I put these together, how many will I have?' He counted: 'Two and another two is four.' He lined them up a different way and counted: 'Two and two is four, bring me the bananas, Ugg!' It worked and works every single time. It is the truth.

We can have faith knowing that gravity is there, two plus two equals four, heat rises, the sun will rise and then set, if you break the law you will get punished, if you save your money you will have more, if you eat well you will be healthy. These are not just crazy ideas. These are laws of the universe and they represent truth and what will happen predictably every single time.

If you can take the time to understand and believe some of the more intangible laws of the universe, having faith becomes an easier position to take. When you can trust things happen predictably, it removes the uncertainty, the fear and the stress. It makes life a more exciting and purpose-driven place. It certainly helps me to live a better life with the faith that everything happens for a reason and everything leads me in the direction I need to go, and that my destiny is secure. I hope that understanding and having faith in these laws of the universe does the same for you.

The law of growth

In a movie called *Evan Almighty*, the actor Steve Carell plays Evan Baxter, a successful newscaster who wins a seat in congress. As a result, he has to uproot his family and move to a new neighbourhood and take advantage of this new opportunity. It takes much of his time, and as a result he starts to compromise and sacrifice time with his family. After many disappointments and frustrations, his wife prays for more family time.

Not long after that, God, in the form of Morgan Freeman, appears and commands Evan to build an ark in preparation for a flood. I won't go into a lot of detail, except to say that all of a sudden Evan has pairs of animals following him down the street and into congress. He starts growing a long white flowing beard and wearing an ancient gown. Despite his confusion and resistance, he soon realises he has no choice but to build the ark, so he gets started.

You're probably wondering where I'm going with this, so bear with me! Evan's wife Joan and children don't understand; they think he's going crazy. At one point, worried about Evan's sanity and scared for their safety, Joan takes the children and leaves. Not long after that she is sitting in a café looking sad, when her waiter comes over and asks if there is anything wrong. She looks up and it's God in the form of a waiter at the café.

She explains that all she wants is a happy family and to spend more quality time together, but that her husband has gone a bit crazy. She explains that she has prayed for a better situation, but it seems to be getting worse. God then asks her: 'If you pray for courage, do you think God gives you courage or an opportunity to show courage?' Joan answers: 'An opportunity to show courage.' He then asks: 'When you pray for knowledge, do you think God gives you that knowledge or an opportunity to learn?' Joan answers: 'An opportunity to learn.'

'Right,' says God, 'so when you pray for a closer family unit, do you think God gives you what you pray for or an opportunity to become closer as a family?' This question impacts Joan and she looks up to find that God has disappeared, but the penny has dropped. Joan and the children returned home to help Evan with the ark, and the movie ends predictably. I love that particular scene.

What's my point? No matter what situation you find yourself in or how undesirable it may seem, it's happening for a reason. It's either a lesson you need to learn, an opportunity for growth or a test to see how committed you are to your goal or aspiration. This is the law that states *everything happens for a reason*.

The scene out of *Evan Almighty* shows that, in this particular case, the situation was an opportunity for a stronger and closer family unit. If you are having health, relationship or financial issues, it's often an indication of something needing to change. It's a lesson you need to learn, or it will keep being presented to you in progressively more extreme circumstances. What about the unexplained or seemingly unlucky thing that happens to challenge you just as you have set yourself a goal or aspiration? That, my friend, is a test to see how serious you are about your goals or dreams.

I made a decision to write the story of my mother's life, cancer journey and the inspiring lessons I learned from her in late September 2004 when I was away with her and my dad on a family holiday in Queensland. I had a wonderful week with her, talking to her and learning about her life, her struggles and her 16-year journey with cancer. At the end of the week I loved her even more (if that was possible), was even more compelled by her and was totally committed to writing a book to share her story and inspire many people all around the world. Soon after that week I was seriously tested!

The first and most devastating test occurred only a couple of months later when my beautiful mother passed away, on 3 December 2004. I was crushed. I'd had 16 years to come to terms with the fact that she may die early, but not for one second did I even consider it an option. I had my head firmly buried far too deeply in the sand. You know what's sticking up to be kicked when your head is in the sand, don't you? Yep; mine was kicked and kicked hard. It took me years to get over the tragic loss.

I was now even more committed to writing a book. I grieved, healed, and was finally ready to move on. I started writing again, and finally in 2008 I proudly finished the manuscript. I sent it to my publishers at the time, expecting the rest of the process would be a simple one. Then came test number two: my publishers rejected the manuscript and said they were not interested in publishing it. I was floored. What do I do now? I did all I knew to do, and started googling publishers and literary agents and sending out submissions.

Test number three was the battle in my own mind. I sent out 40 to 50 manuscripts and received rejection after rejection after rejection! There were so many times it felt hopeless and I felt like giving up, but then I thought about my mother – her courage, her resilience and her determination – and needless to say I kept going. The burn inside me was strong. I knew it would happen, I just didn't know it would take so long.

Finally, in late 2009, the manuscript was accepted by a publisher and I was excited ... until I was tested yet again. I received an email from the editor, which started in a positive way. She said: 'Well, my brain has done its thinking and I've put some very rough ideas down for how I think the manuscript and general approach needs to be reworked.' She ended the same email with: 'I'll leave the feedback there for now as that's quite a lot for you to take in! Hopefully I haven't shocked you into depression!'

I wasn't depressed. I was, however, intimidated and overwhelmed by the confronting changes I needed to make. But I had a dream, so I got to work and reworked, rewrote and reformatted a large part of the manuscript. Finally, in February 2011, almost seven years later, I received my first published copy of *Dance Until It Rains*. It was a proud and exciting moment. It was a tribute to my beautiful mother. It was her legacy. It was a burning desire. I'm sure you can see that, no matter how I was tested over those seven long years, I was always going to find a way to overcome my challenges because the goal was strong and the decision to get it done had been made. I had faith!

The law of attraction

You've heard it said before in many different ways: what you sow, so shall you reap. What you give, you will get. It's a powerful law of the universe: the law of reciprocity, the law of karma, the law of attraction; call it whatever you want. It's there, it's happening and it's affecting your life whether you know it, believe it, or like it or not.

Whatever you are getting in your life you are attracting through this powerful law. Why do some people seem to have all the luck and others seem to have no luck? How do some people make friends easily and others seem to have one conflict after another? Why do some people seem to have all the time and money they need while others never seem to have enough of either? What you give will come back, often in abundance! Let's start with a couple of simple examples. If you smile at someone today, what will happen? Yes; they will smile back at you. If you are angry at someone because of something they did or said and angrily blame them for your problems, what will happen? Will they smile, hug you and give you some money? In your dreams!! They will either snap back at you or they will get away from you as quickly as possible. What you give out you will get back.

I stopped to get some healthy food for lunch recently. I smiled at and started chatting to the guy serving me and I asked him about his day. I complimented him on the job he was doing, then after I'd paid for my food he offered me a free sample of one of their products. Was it luck, or because he was a nice person? I think I'm blessed, not lucky, and I do believe he was a very nice person. But would he have given me that free sample if I didn't give him friendliness and a compliment? I doubt it. What if I'd gone in, demanded food, waited impatiently and insulted him for taking too long: would I have received a free sample? No chance. In fact, he may have added something not quite as savoury into my food!

What you give out you will get back. If you want more time, then give more time. If you want more money, then give more money. If you want more love, then give more love. It's a powerful law of the universe and it will deliver every single time. Back when I was working 80 plus hours per week in my personal training business, and had been for 15 years, I wanted one thing: more time to write books and do things I was passionate about. I made a seemingly crazy decision at that time to invest even more time into another business. This business had the potential to provide me with an asset-based income to buy back some of my time.

With a small investment of five to 10 hours per week outside of my 80 plus–hour fitness business, for the next 10 months I changed my whole deal. I developed a business that produced an ongoing income to enable me to sell my personal training business back to my partner and stop working evenings. I went from working 80 hours per week to 30 hours per week. In other words, I gave up five to 10 hours per week for 10 months and in return I received an extra 50 hours per week to do with as I chose. I chose more time with my wife, more time for myself and more time to become a full-time author. What you give out will come back in abundance. Have faith in this law of the universe.

The law of perspective

Enjoy this story ...

Many centuries ago lived a king and his loyal servant. They were inseparable, and the servant pandered to every need of the king. As diligent and attentive as the servant was, he did have one slightly annoying habit. No matter what the situation, the servant would always say 'This is good'. It irritated the king a little, but because his servant was so loyal he would regularly let it pass.

One day the king decided to go hunting and instructed his servant to fetch and pack his gun. What neither of them realised was that the servant had incorrectly packed the gun. As a result of the error made by the servant, when the king went to fire his gun he blew off his thumb. The king stood there in excruciating pain, with blood spurting out of the place where his thumb had been. The servant's response was predictable: 'This is good.'

Clearly this did not please the king. In fact, it angered him even more. He ordered his servant back to the castle, then had him locked away. He was chained by his ankles upside down in the deepest dungeon and hung there for the next 12 months.

A year later the king, minus one thumb, decided to go hunting again. This time he packed his own gun and double checked that it was done correctly. He left the castle on his own to hunt wild animals, but no sooner was he in the forest when he was captured by cannibals. They placed him a large cauldron of water on an open fire to kill him and then offer him as a sacrifice to their god.

Just as the king was about to perish, the cannibals noticed he was missing a thumb. He was no longer a worthy sacrifice and they released him.

The king jumped on his horse, raced back to the castle, ran down to the deepest dungeon and released his servant. As soon as the servant was on two feet and coherent, the king said: 'You were right, losing my thumb was good.' Then he added: 'And what I did to you was bad!' The servant replied: 'No, no, that was good. If I wasn't in this dungeon, I would have been with you!'

What a wonderfully entertaining illustration of how we can find good in every situation. It's all how we look at things. If you can have faith in knowing that no matter what happens in your life some good will come from it, then you will have a positive perspective about every situation, whether on the surface it seems good or bad. I can tell you from my own personal experience I am a calmer, more peaceful and, ultimately, healthier person as a result of this universal law.

The law of choice

One of the definitions of faith is: 'Faith is seeing light with your heart when all your eyes see is darkness.' When we see darkness, adversity or problems we usually follow that by choosing to respond with a corresponding thought that leads to an emotion such as sadness, anger, guilt, resentment, fear, jealousy, frustration, grief, despair, doubt or one of the many other negative and destructive emotions. Yes, I said *we choose*! This is truth.

We cannot hold two opposing emotions in our bodies at the same time. In other words, we can't be happy and sad at the same time. We can't be resentful and grateful at the same time. We can't be depressed and excited at the same time. We can't be angry and loving at the same time. This is also truth.

If it is true you get to choose the thoughts that lead to your emotional response and it is also true you can't hold two opposing feelings in your body at the same time, then that means you can very easily trade one feeling for another feeling. As soon as you start to notice a negative and destructive emotion, quickly trade if for another positive thought and feeling. When you feel resentment rising in your body because your partner is nagging you, immediately trade it for gratitude that they care enough to say anything. What else do you have to be grateful for? Whenever you feel anger towards someone starting to boil, think instantly of what you love about that person. Whenever you feel fear rearing its ugly head, swap it for the excitement you'll feel when you've achieved the task that is causing the fear. Have faith, knowing at any moment you can trade and choose the feeling that will bring health and happiness into your life.

The law of the path

If you travel, you will know that once you are on the proper trajectory and keep going you will predictably arrive at your desired destination, right? If, however, your intention is to get to Sydney, Australia and you get on a plane that has a flight heading towards Perth, Australia, your intention is irrelevant; you are going to Perth! That sounds so obvious, doesn't it? I mean, who would possibly get on a plane heading one way with a logical intention to head in the opposite direction?

That's an interesting question to ponder. As crazy as it may seem to head in the wrong direction – and I don't know about you – but I do it far too often. Have you ever had a good intention to create a better relationship with your partner and then criticised them or argued with them about something silly? Wrong direction! Have you ever set the intention to get leaner and look after your health and then, because you were busy, drove through a popular fast food outlet for a convenient meal? Wrong direction! Have you ever decided to improve your financial position and then spontaneously purchased the newest high-tech flat screen television because no one else you knew had one and it fitted that space on the wall perfectly? Wrong direction!

Do you get what I'm saying? Your intention is irrelevant; it's the decisions you make and the direction you take that will determine your destination. This is predictable, so there is no need to be surprised when your relationship falters, your health fails and your financial situation plummets. It was the predictable outcome of the actions you were choosing and the path you were on. This is described brilliantly by the pastor of North Point Church in Atlanta, Georgia, Andy Stanley, in his book *The Principle of the Path*. Andy says very clearly that it's your *direction*, not *your intention*, that will determine your destination. Just so you know, this is very good news!

This means you can have faith in the fact that if you make the right decisions, take the appropriate actions and persist, you will inevitably and reliably achieve your desired result. Remember the quote by Philip Yancey: 'Faith is believing in advance what only makes sense in reverse.' If you have faith and take the right actions, you will look back and see how much sense it made.

If you decide to eat a healthy breakfast every day, and you do it *every day*, you will be leaner, healthier and more energised and you will make better eating choices throughout the day. This is predictable. If you put money into savings every week, and do it every week, you won't have to cross your fingers in the hope you will be financially secure. It will be inevitable. If you do something loving and/or respectful of your partner every single day, and don't miss a day, your relationship will be happy, strong and blissful. You can count on that.

I am writing this section of this book at the moment, but at the time you're reading this it has obviously been written, finished and published. Why? It is because I clearly keep my intention and my direction consistent. I know that writing a book is simple: if I write a little every day and commit to keep going, then I don't have to cross my fingers and hope it will get done. I have faith with every book I write that, while my intention is to have a best-selling published book, I know it is my daily activity that sets my direction and it's my direction that will determine my destination.

The law of intuition

Have you ever noticed an unsettling feeling in the pit of your stomach when you make certain decisions, then not long afterwards you experience an undesirable outcome of some sort? Alternatively, have you ever felt strong, in control and in a flow, like things were happening easily and everything seems to be going as you want? This is your intuition – your internal guidance system – and it will always lead you in the right direction if you listen to and follow it. The problem for many people is that they ignore it or override it, and then suffer the consequences down the track.

Your intuition is directed by your values. Every time you make decisions that align with and complement your values, you will flow into a positive outcome. For that you can have faith. On the other hand, whenever you act in conflict with your values you will feel it in the pit of your stomach. If you continue to act in spite of this internal warning it will end badly, trust me.

You will be able to come up with many examples that illustrate both ends of the spectrum. Let me give you two that highlight the incredible power of going with your intuition and the devastating error in judgement if you don't. We all make poorly considered decisions in our lives and we all ignore that gut feeling at times, don't we? I have done it more times than I'm willing to share with you, except this one.

I was at a stage in my life when I had come out of a failed café which, for two years, had taken my life and all of my money, and I was trying to recover myself financially, physically and emotionally. Not long after that, as I was getting back on my feet and no longer worried about sleeping in the streets, I was introduced through a mutual friend to a guy who sold investments. I wanted to get financially strong again, and I wanted to do it quickly! Ever tried that? Bad move, hey? I sat with this guy, who showed me the potential return on my investment, which was significant. I was momentarily blinded by the sparkling shiny object in front of me. I was so blinded that I didn't pay attention to the uneasy feeling in my gut.

I signed the papers. I committed a significant amount of money each month that I didn't have, and within 12 months the investment bombed and I was further into the financial toilet! Hindsight is a wonderful thing. We can all look back and see the error in our choices, can't we? However, no longer do we need to rely on learning through hindsight if we can become aware of that intuitive gut feeling that is always there and actually listen to it. You will save yourself much heartbreak, poverty and despair.

When you do listen to it – oh, my goodness – the whole world will open up to you and for you. The craziest, the most illogical decision I ever made was to become an author. At the time I was working in two businesses, for 12 to 15 hours seven days per week. I have a football background, struggled to pass English at high school, rarely read and never once, until that moment, had any aspiration to write anything, let alone a book! So why would I possibly come to the conclusion that writing a book would be a good idea, other than my intuition?

I don't know how, but I found pockets of time and just two years after that irrational decision I had written two best-selling books. From that moment and until this day, I can look back and see that everything great that has happened to me and for me was the result of the one simple, unreasonable and unlikely decision. From that point my life has been in a flow and I know I live an incredible life of passion. Why? Because I went with my intuition, not my logic.

The law of intuition will work for you as it will for me and every person on the planet. Have faith that when you listen to that gut feeling it will keep you in line with your values and direct you to choices that will enable you to live an amazing life of abundance, joy and passion.

Putting the pieces in place

I'm not sure how you reacted to this chapter or whether you can see how it fits as one of the crucial pieces of the wellness puzzle. What I will say to you from my perspective, is that the moment I was able to have faith and believe in what I couldn't see my life started to change for the better. Again, I refer back to that spontaneous decision I made to write a book – wow! It was faith, certainly not logic or prior experience, that has led me to this point in my life.

I now know that happiness and well-being are outcomes. They are the result of the peace of mind that comes from having faith in a higher purpose. It happens when you know you are on the path and you are being led to where you need to be. It's the consequence of trusting the powerful laws of the universe or the scriptures of the Bible.

I want to encourage you to just have faith, even if what I'm talking about in this chapter is confronting for you. What do you have to lose? For just a short time, give up the need for being in control, for validation from external sources and for thinking luck has anything to do with outcomes in your life. Feel the peace that comes from having faith that everything is going to be okay.

Close your eyes, take a couple of deep breaths in and feel the security that comes from knowing you are on the right path and are being led in the direction you ultimately want to go. There are many stories of people who found themselves in troubled times, but with faith have been able to move on to a place of wellness, significance, purpose and abundance. The same will happen to you as soon as you have faith.

 ## Key questions and action steps

1. Can you think of instances in your life when just having faith was the right decision?

2. Can you see how having faith will give you the peace of mind of knowing you are on the right path and all you need for a happy life is already there for you?

3. Each day, take yourself to a quiet place and sit for a few minutes with your eyes closed. Breathe deeply and feel the calmness that comes with an inner knowing that you are being divinely and/or universally led.

4. While you are sitting with your eyes closed each day, forgive yourself for things you are beating yourself up over and make

a fresh start, knowing that your past is not your future and you can create any outcome you desire.

5. Even if it's difficult for you, start to believe in, practise and have faith in the universal laws that I touched on.

6. The law of growth: with every seemingly undesirable situation you are facing or will face, ask yourself: is this a lesson, a test or an opportunity for growth? Each situation will help you become better, stronger and wiser.

7. The law of attraction: everything you think, do or say will come back to you. Have faith that if you put out positive thoughts, words and actions they will come back to help you in your life. Understand and be aware that the opposite is also true.

8. The law of perspective: find the good in every situation; it is there if you look for it.

9. The law of choice: you can't hold two opposing thoughts or emotions in your mind and body at the same time. Whenever you have a negative thought and emotion, quickly trade it for a positive one.

10. The law of the path: have faith that every eventuality is the predictable result of your daily actions, which will determine your direction. Make sure you take the actions that will lead you where you want to go.

11. The law of intuition: trust your gut feeling and go with it!

Move your body
One step at a time

It's not just about the steps or the distance: it's about the mindset and habit you will create. Every decision will move you closer to optimal well-being or further away. There is no middle ground or plateau point.

How good does it feel when you finally get to the last piece of a puzzle? With ease and pride, you slide it in as you feel the satisfaction that comes from knowing you have finished what you started. You have successfully completed the puzzle and have the beautiful picture in front of you. Well, we are at that stage in your wellness puzzle.

If you are still with me reading this chapter, then I will assume you are paying attention to, and have started to make some changes to, putting the first six pieces of the puzzle in place. That being the case, you should be feeling amazing. Am I right? What I can tell you now is that if you have started working on the first six pieces, this last one is a piece of cake (pardon the pun).

Aaaagghh: exercise! You either love it or hate it, prioritise it or avoid it, have made a habit of doing it or have come up with a raft of excuses why you can't. The bottom line is, no matter your attitude towards exercise, you cannot and will not be optimally healthy without developing a habit and regime of movement in your life. You knew that already though, didn't you?

I'm not going to spend too much time nor insult your intelligence by going into details of all the benefits of regular exercise, except to say one thing. If you want to look and feel amazing, feel good about yourself, have more self-confidence, get through your day with ease, live a longer, more fulfilling and productive life, achieve some of the ambitious goals you've set for yourself, have the energy to spend time with people you care about, do things that are important to you, set a positive example for your family and be in the very small percentage of people who are optimally healthy, then, exercise is a non-negotiable price you will need to pay.

Now, trust me on this one: it's not the price you are maybe thinking of. It doesn't mean you have to exercise two hours per day, seven days per week. It doesn't require the pain and suffering that many people believe is necessary. It doesn't require a large financial investment. It doesn't need to be a chore or a sacrifice. Moving your body just needs to become a daily habit.

My introduction to the world of exercise was an extreme one. At the age of 16, I was invited to go and train for a professional Australian football club, the St Kilda Saints. I gladly accepted the invitation in anticipation of a glamorous and exciting football career. I can tell you that my excitement turned into agony within only a few minutes of my very first training session. The following text is from my book about my football career:

I clearly remember my very first training session at the St Kilda Football Club. I was young and naïve, it was a beautiful Saturday morning in September 1980 and the entire under nineteen's squad met at the beach for what I thought would be a pleasant introductory ten kilometre (six mile) run. I expected that we would just be cruising along the picturesque track at the top of the cliff, enjoying the beautiful coastal scenery. Boy, did I get it wrong. There are many words I could use to describe that session, 'cruising' is not one of them.

We started running, at a disturbingly fast pace, and not too far along the track we took a detour which didn't look good. We ran down a steep ramp and onto the beach. The morning was hot, the sand was soft and the competition was fierce. I didn't think it was a race, but what I came to realise very quickly was, at a professional football club when there were only twenty-two spots in the senior team and over one hundred players vying for them, everything was a competition!

Running through soft sand on a hot day is bad enough. Running through soft sand on a hot day with other players trying to knock you over and slow you down is another thing altogether. We ran along the sand for what seemed to be an eternity and then we came to another steep ramp. It was great to put my feet on solid ground despite the fact that my legs felt like jelly. The relief was short lived as we had to immediately run up this long and steep ramp. I have never experienced so much agony in my life.

When we got to the top I almost collapsed, but somehow kept going and, over the next few minutes, was able to recover just enough to reach the next ramp which took us back down to the beach to do it all over again. This stretch of sand was longer, softer and more torturous than before. The good news was that the beach was coming to an end with no ramp in sight. All I could see was a fifty-metre vertical cliff ... there was no way out. Surely that meant we would have to stop.

No such luck! We got to the bottom of this seemingly unassailable cliff and were instructed to climb it! I was shattered and on the verge of giving up. My legs were rubber, my lungs were on fire and I could see no physical way I could get to the top. Then, from behind, I heard *'come on Jobbas, you can do it.'* Some encouragement, finally! It was so welcomed, it spurred me on and with it I dug deeper to somehow claw my way to the top of the cliff.

I fell over at the top and then crawled on hands and knees for a while until I somehow got back up onto my feet and stumbled down the road the final kilometre and fell across the finish line. I honestly don't know if I would've made it to the top of the cliff or the end of the run without those few words of encouragement.

Welcome to the big league sooky boy! Clearly, it was a rough introduction to the life of a professional sportsman. I was initially focused on the fame, the fortune and the glamour. In no way had I prepared myself for the reality of this life. Ninety per cent of the time over the next seven years is easily summed up in one word — PAIN!

This was my grounding and attitude development for exercise from a young age, and I can tell you it's been both a blessing and a curse at the same time. Consequently, I have a love-hate relationship with exercise – a hangover from my professional sporting days. I hated doing it because it hurt so much, but I loved it when it was over because it had enabled me to achieve the things I wanted. Even today, many years later, I have a similar attitude towards exercise: I don't look forward to it, but I love the feeling when I'm finished and I'm absolutely addicted to how I look and feel as a result.

I certainly don't believe people need to exercise at a high intensity unless they have a serious fitness or sporting aspiration. I do, however, think the challenge most have in sticking to an exercise regime is *focus* – they are focusing on the wrong thing. Have you ever set your alarm with the intention of getting up early to exercise? Have you then woken up to the alarm, thought about that intention, hit the snooze button and gone back to sleep? Remember it is your direction, not your intention, that determines your destination!

I think we've all done that, haven't we? When I've hit the snooze before it's because, rather than focusing on how good I'll feel after I get myself up and finish my exercise session, I think about how hard it is to get up and how uncomfortable exercising will be. I very quickly and easily talk myself out of it. Do you relate to what I'm saying? These days, I get up every time I set my alarm to exercise and not because I'm anything special; let me be clear on that one. It's because I have one thought in my mind and one thought only: the end! I visualise how amazing and proud I will feel when I'm finished. I think about the benefit it will have on my mind and body. I think about my vision to live to one hundred years old and how important that session really is. I think about my desire to want to be healthy, fit and energised all my life. The result is that every day when my alarm goes off, without any further procrastination, I get up.

Step one in the process of moving your body is to get sold on to the amazing benefits of exercise and how it will help you achieve your purpose in life. Every single time focus on how good you'll feel when you've finished, not how uncomfortable it will be. Now, don't get me wrong; it may be uncomfortable at times, but if that is what you think, then the chances of making excuses are far greater. When you think about your purpose, when you focus on the reasons why exercise will help you in your life, you will stop negotiating the price and do it with enthusiasm and energy.

The biggest mistake I made when I was starting out as a personal trainer – fresh from seven years of regular and ongoing pain as a professional footballer – was the incorrect assumption that exercise had to be hard and painful and lead to exhaustion if it were to be effective. It was all I knew. After several injuries, vomiting clients, regular no-shows and too many cancellations I had enough sense to question what I was doing. It was then I realised that most people don't want to be professional athletes. Instead, they want to be lean and healthy and enjoy their lives. At that time I was just another source of stress for them, so I changed my approach.

I actually listened to my clients and surprise, surprise, I even found out what they wanted. I was able to help them develop an exercise plan that suited them, their goals and their personal circumstances. I paid more attention to their nutrition, as I've already discussed in previous chapters. I transformed myself from the tyrant trainer who was always trying to inflict pain – maybe as a payback from all the pain inflicted on me – to one who genuinely wanted to help my clients create good habits and get great results. My biggest challenge, even with my more moderate and friendly approach, was keeping clients on track.

Is it time to get off your excuse?

Even with a strong reason, a desire to change and a commitment to an exercise regime we can get swayed to the dark side, can't we? No matter who you are, what you do and what you want, you are going to get impacted by the three Ds at some stage: **d**oubt, **d**iscouragement and **d**istraction. It doesn't matter whether you are just walking each day to keep moving or training like a maniac for a serious fitness goal, we are all human and all vulnerable at times.

When you feel any of the three Ds start to impact, you need to refocus back on your big picture and the reason you're exercising in the first place. In addition to that, you need to be able to get yourself back up, off your excuse and into action again, whether you feel like it or want to or not. You need to rely less on motivation and more on doing it anyway. In my thirty years in the health and fitness industry, I have heard pretty much every excuse under the sun. While each excuse may have some validity and be justifiable, it is never helpful.

I know in advance what you would say to me if I was training you and you felt doubtful, discouraged and/or distracted. In fact, I'm going to tell you. Not only that, I'm going to help you move past each and every challenge, problem, excuse or whatever you want to call it. I'm going to list the top 20 excuses I've heard and I'm going to dispel them. Not to be insensitive, not to be un-empathetic, but to help you make better choices. Remember this: you can be optimally healthy *or* make excuses; you can't do both!

Excuse 1: I can't be bothered and am not motivated.
Solution: stop relying on motivation – it is unreliable – and do it anyway. Very soon action and exercise will become a habit. Getting started requires you

to think about and get emotionally connected to your 'why?' If the exercise doesn't motivate you, will your family, your life and/or your own success do it?

Excuse 2: I don't enjoy it.

Solution: many people, including myself, don't enjoy it. Will you enjoy the feeling of getting it done? Will you enjoy looking and feeling great? Will you enjoy quality time with your family? Will you enjoy your increased productivity? Will you enjoy more energy and a happier life? You don't need to enjoy it, you just need to do it! Having said that, could you try and find a sport or activity that you do enjoy?

Excuse 3: it hurts.

Solution: yes, it can hurt at times. Focus on the benefits and your dreams, not on the uncomfortable process.

Excuse 4: I don't know what I should be doing.

Solution: find someone who can help you and listen to them.

Excuse 5: it's too expensive.

Solution: it costs nothing except the investment in a good pair of shoes and some training gear to go for a walk or run, do some step ups, climb some stairs or find a park to do some strength exercises. It just takes a decision.

Excuse 6: I'm too tired.

Solution: that's all the more reason to get started on your exercise regime. Start small and build up progressively. Make sure you are eating to fuel your body. Tiredness is often a state of mind and a result of your self-talk. Start telling yourself you are full of energy, and guess what will happen?

Excuse 7: it's too hot.

Solution: go swimming.

Excuse 8: it's too cold.

Solution: rug up, and when you're warm disrobe. Alternatively, train inside at a gym, to an exercise video or an in-home program.

Excuse 9: it's raining.

Solution: get wet, you are waterproof. Refer to the solution for excuse 8.

Excuse 10: it's too windy.

Solution: I think you know what to do here.

Excuse 11: I've no one to exercise with.

Solution: do it alone and you will soon inspire someone to exercise with you.

Excuse 12: I've no support, and get negative reactions.

Solution: this can be a difficult one and I'm going to say something that may seem insensitive, for which I make no apologies: toughen up! Think about whose dream, whose life, whose well-being it is anyway. Remember that any lack of support or negativity is coming from people who are thinking of themselves, not you. Don't allow them to steal your dream for optimal well-being. Be strong, courageous and determined. In fact, you will be amazed how those same people will start to support you when they see how serious you are and committed to your desire to change.

Excuse 13: I don't see any results.

Solution: be patient, as there is no quick fix or easy answer; it will take time. It often depends on you, your body, your mindset, your stress levels and your metabolism. If you take positive, responsible and consistent action with a suitable plan and stick to it you will predictably get the results you want.

Excuse 14: I'm bored with exercise.

Solution: really? Will you be bored with being fit, lean and healthy? Again, it's simply a matter of changing your focus to the results and benefits you will achieve rather than the process. If boredom is that much of a problem, find an exercise that doesn't bore you; there are so many things you can do. This excuse is really just a cop-out.

Excuse 15: I have sore legs or a leg injury.
Solution: get creative and find upper body exercises you can do that don't bother your legs.

Excuse 16: I have sore arms or an upper body injury.
Solution: find lower body exercises you can do that don't bother your upper body. What about walking?

Excuse 17: I have lower back issues.
Solution: welcome to the club; so do most people. I have had lower back issues for most of my life. Through proper management, regular movement and strengthening of your core muscles, this should not be a barrier. There is always something you can do; your job is to find it and do it.

Excuse 18: I have health issues.
Solution: oh, my gosh, if there is any reason to commit to an appropriate exercise regime, that is it. Let it be your reason, not your excuse … if you want to get better, that is.

Excuse 19: I have no time and am too busy.
Solution: if you can't choose to find time for your health and fitness now, you will be forced to find time to recover lost health in the future. You are not too busy and you do have time; you just haven't given exercise enough of a priority in your life. If you don't have 60 minutes four times per week, find 30 minutes four times per week. If you can't do that, find 15 minutes five times per week. If that's too hard, find five minutes each day. If you can't do that, you're not trying or serious about your well-being.

Excuse 20: Anything else.

Solution: focus on what you want, get over yourself, find a solution and get it done!

The good news is that we have now removed pretty much any and every excuse you may have to get started on a regular and ongoing exercise regime. This chapter is less about telling you exactly what you should be doing and more about helping you commit to doing something. There are many great books, resources, experts, gyms and personal trainers out there ready to help you find what's right for you. At this moment, if exercise is your missing puzzle piece it only takes a decision. The first step is to forget about finishing and focus on starting.

Creating optimal well-being, one step at a time

Let's start with a foundational and simple baseline decision, then go from there. This is somewhere we can all start from no matter our age, our circumstances, our goals or our physical condition. Just start walking and commit to it every single day. If you have some type of physical limitation to walking don't let that be your excuse; find some other simple foundational movement you can commit to each day. For the rest of us, if we walk every day, measure our steps and don't go to bed until we've achieved the number of steps we've committed to, it's amazing what will happen.

'Honestly, is walking of any real value and benefit? It seems too easy.' This was a question I asked myself regularly. As you already know, I was an all-or-nothing, no-pain-no-gain, go-hard-or-go-home kinda guy. I would trash myself in training for at least an hour each day and then be a slob for the rest of the day. I thought I'd done enough and deserved it. I laughed at people who strapped on their pedometer or Fitbit and obsessively tracked their steps for the day. Oh, how clueless I was!

As you may know, it is strongly recommended in wellness circles that we aim for at least 10,000 steps per day. I laughed and thought I easily nailed it by 9 am each day. How wrong I was. When I finally started measuring my steps to prove how easily I was achieving the target, I was horrified to discover that I only averaged about 5,000 steps each day. My first reaction was that the pedometer didn't work, then I justified it by convincing myself that the training I did made up for the shortfall of steps. I finally slapped myself, got over my ego and got committed to doing 10,000 steps every day. As a result my thinking and attitude changed, my mindset changed, my habits changed, my physical condition changed and my life changed. It will for you also.

Think about this to blow your mind: before my commitment to 10,000 steps per day I was averaging 5,000 steps. Walking the extra 5,000 steps at an average pace would take about 30 to 45 minutes, and it could be spread out over the course of the day – it didn't have to be done in one go. So, it's not that big a deal or major effort. If I convert my steps to distance, 5,000 steps translate to three and a half kilometres (just over two miles). Again, that's really no big deal, is it? It would even be easy to think that it's an insignificant distance and to talk myself out of it. I could easily justify that by saying 'it's only a small distance and it won't matter if I miss a day here or there'.

It's true in one day it's not a large distance, but what if I commit to doing it every day? (I have.) I now walk an extra 1,300 kilometres (807 miles) every year. To give this some perspective, it's the approximate distance of walking from Sydney, New South Wales to Adelaide, South Australia in Australia, from New York, New York to Atlanta, Georgia in the USA and from Paris, France to Vienna, Austria in Europe. It sounds undo-able, doesn't it? It sounds unrealistic and far fetched, but it's very possible when broken down to a little bit every day. Do you think you would be fitter, leaner and healthier if you walked an extra 1,300 kilometres per year? You bet you would!

It's not just about the steps or the distance; it's very much about the mindset and habit you will create. Every decision will move you closer to optimal well-being or further away. There is no middle ground or plateau point. You are either flying or falling, succeeding or failing, strengthening or eroding, building or destroying. It sounds dramatic, doesn't it? It is, so be very careful about every decision you make. It's so easy to track your steps and walk that little extra each day, but it's even easier not to.

Each choice you make will strengthen, reinforce and build the mindset that will lead to a habit. When you choose to hit your 10,000 steps for the day and you do it regardless of how you feel or whatever time of the day it requires, you are strengthening the mindset and habit that will lead to optimal health. If you justify to yourself that you've had a busy day, you're too tired, you'll do the extra tomorrow and that it's no big deal, you are strengthening the mindset and habit that will lead to ongoing frustration, failure and physical imbalance.

It took me a while to really understand the power of 10,000 steps per day, and now I don't allow myself to go to bed until it is done. In fact, I have recently increased my target to 12,000 steps and have a sign next to my bed that says, 'If you haven't done your 12,000, start stepping!' I can tell you for a fact that you only need to leave it to the last minute a few times before you get organised enough to make sure it's done by bedtime. There have been several occasions when, at 11 pm, Laura has been yelling at me, 'What's that stomping sound? What are you doing?' It's me doing my last few thousand steps so I can finally go to bed!

Thanks goodness for my ole dinosaur of a pedometer; it's the best tool I know of to help create this wonderful habit. You may have one or you may have some other sort of high-tech measuring tool. Either way, can I suggest you get yourself some device that measures your daily steps? There is a saying: what you measure will improve. If you know how many steps you do, you can set tangible and effective goals for yourself. For me, my pedometer is an incredibly powerful motivator. It keeps me on track and it holds me accountable for doing my twelve thousand steps each day.

I want to help you with this and share with you some ideas for establishing this non-negotiable foundation of fitness. If you can understand and believe that doing at least 10,000 steps every day is a key to your well-being and helping you follow your passion in life and purpose for being, you are more likely to take it seriously. As I mentioned earlier, once this foundation is in place and you are enjoying the benefits – physical, emotional and mental – of your daily habit, you will be more inspired and motivated to layer additional exercise strategies on top of it. This is where true fitness and wellness benefits will start to flow to you.

I've learned the hard way from too many nights of jogging on the spot at 11 pm that the best option is to get my 12,000 steps done, or as near to done as possible, as early in the day as I can. My routine is my routine and I'm only telling you about it to help you come up with your own. I am known to do some strange stuff, but then, I like being strange. I like doing what many people would probably not do, and I like being, looking and feeling the way I do as a result. What about you?

I get up between 5.30 am and 6 am each day with the exception of the weekend, when it may be an hour later. I attach my pedometer and do my necessities, which include my affirmations while looking at myself in the mirror. I'm of the attitude that if I can maximise my time and do two things at once then I'll do it. This for a man with limited multitasking skills is impressive to me. While I'm standing in the bathroom looking in the mirror and affirming positive statements I jog on the spot. I may as well get some steps done at the same time!

I then do my exercise session, which lasts from 30 to 60 minutes and is a variety of different types of cardiovascular exercise and resistance training. By the end of that session I have usually done between 4,000 and 5,000 steps. So far this is nothing that unusual, right? Then I take my two fluffy four-legged kids for a 20-minute walk. Again, this is nothing out of the ordinary, is it?

My theory is if I'm going to be walking my dogs anyway and if it's going to take 20 minutes, I may as well get as many steps as I can in that time. If I walk with them, stopping when they stop, I will do about 1,500 steps. If, however, I jog on the spot at all times, including when they stop to sniff, wee and poo, I can do 3,000 to 4,000 steps in that same 20 minutes.

Most people get frustrated when their dogs stop and sniff at every single tree; I encourage it. The more they stop to do what dogs do, the more steps I get. Yes, I look weird and yes, people often look at me and laugh. Just ask the workmen on the construction site that I pass every morning how weird I look. They stare at me every morning as I go past and they talk among themselves. I can imagine exactly what they are saying, and it's nothing complimentary I'm sure. At least I am a source of their daily amusement, but I don't care. By 7.30 am most mornings I have done around 8,000 steps, and I find that it's quite easy to do the remining steps by the end of the day.

Doing 10,000 steps every day is simple if you pay attention. There are so many wonderful opportunities from the second you get up to the moment you go to bed to add steps to your daily tally. Jogging on the spot, whenever you can, is one of them. Do you really care what other people think? Walking around while you're on the phone is easy. Taking your dog, cat, kids, friend and/or partner for a walk is an obvious step-increasing activity. Not so obvious are all the other benefits that go with it: relationship building, time out of your stressful day and the powerful habit you are creating.

When you drive to the shopping centre and you are circling as you look for a car park, if you're not measuring your steps, which spot do you want? The closest one, right? If you have your pedometer or Fitbit and are committed to 10,000 steps, which car park will you look for? You will actively look for the one on the outskirts of the parking area, won't you? Isn't it crazy how we circle around and around for 10 to 15 minutes trying to find the closest possible car park, when there are hundreds available that simply require a short walk to the centre?

What about when you're in the shopping centre and you have to go up a level? You will often be presented with a choice: stairs or escalators. I'm a bit weird, as you've possibly already realised, and I will often sit at the bottom observing people and their choices. Those people who are clearly not measuring and not deliberate about their well-being – which is around 90 per cent of people – switch their brains into neutral, step on the escalator and miss out on one of the best opportunities to add steps to their count and wellness to their lives. I, in fact, have a love-hate relationship with stairs. I hate them because they hurt and love them because they are one of the best ways for me to increase my fitness and well-being. Can you see what a powerful and paradigm-shifting tool your step counting device is?

You can walk more around the house or the office. You can park further away from your destination and walk a bit further. You can get off public transport one stop earlier and walk the rest of the way. You can walk for 10 minutes to the corner store, rather than drive it in two. You can base social activities around walking and talking instead of sitting and eating. You can encourage your children to get off their devices and go outside with you to play sport, have fun at the playground or just enjoy nature. There is no limit to the ways of easily reaching 10,000 steps per day. If it's important to you, if you set the goal and if you decide to make it happen, you will get it done.

Your pedometer or counting device is your friend and will guide you with personal accountability, simple motivation and exact measurement to create an amazingly positive habit, one that will place this final piece of the wellness puzzle into position for you. You can do it, one step at a time. This is the beginning and the foundation of your exercise regime. Make a decision to never again go to bed without having done at least 10,000 steps – or the equivalent if there is a physical barrier to walking for you.

Putting the pieces in place

This is a simple piece to put into the puzzle. It doesn't require research, it doesn't require education, it doesn't require ability, it doesn't require lots of time, it doesn't require a financial investment and it certainly doesn't require all the consternation, procrastination and over-thinking you are possibly giving it. All it requires is a simple decision.

That decision is this: if your purpose in life is important enough, would you be willing to commit to a minimum of 10,000 steps per day? That's it!

Everything else you do from an exercise point of view, and all the results you will get through a daily commitment to move your body, will flow from this ridiculously simple yet life-altering decision. Are you ready to do it?

I want to emphasise this point one more time: the fitness you achieve, the wellness you create and the life you live are the results of simple daily steps. Your fitness will improve, your health can be restored and your body can look and feel amazing, one step at a time! Every single seemingly insignificant step you take adds one to your pedometer or Fitbit, adds a tiny piece to your fitness, establishes a stronger habit, develops a mindset of success, moves you closer to your goal and will improve your life. Yes, every single step!

When you can think about your health and fitness this way, it seems do-able, doesn't it? It removes the intimidation factor of gyms, muscle heads and athletes and allows you to just move in the direction you want to go, one step at a time. Your options from here are; get started, get serious or get ripped and rock hard. It's up to you and it all starts with that one decision to not go to bed until you have done your 10,000 steps.

 ## Key questions and action steps

1. Are you happy with the amount of movement you are currently doing?

2. If nothing changes, how will you be feeling and where will you be in the next five or 10 years?

3. When you think about what's most important to you, does finding a way of doing 10,000 steps per day really seem like that massive a commitment?

4. If you are committed to this process, I say, well done. Do you have a step-measuring device? If not, can you purchase one today?

5. Just one step and one day at a time. Don't allow yourself to end the day on less than 10,000 steps, or whatever goal is appropriate for you.

6. If you need to, find someone to partner with and/or keep you accountable to this goal.

7. Go forth and multiply … your steps, that is!

7

Move your body
Stepping it up

The key to the success of any fitness program is your reason
'why?' Without a strong reason, sticking to it will be more difficult,
especially when the novelty period wears off and discomfort starts
to take its place.

Once you are moving, motivation will come

I want to encourage you to set the goal to move your body every single day. For you, just walking 10,000 steps each day may be enough to achieve your health and well-being goals. If that's the case, then I'm happy if you're happy. The last thing I want to do is try and convince you to train like a maniac just for the sake of it; neither you nor I want to do that. In fact, the benefits of walking go way beyond any muscular and physiological adaptation you will enjoy: it's time out, it's fun, it's social, it's meditative, it's habit forming, it's a mindset developing and it's a motivating platform for anyone who wants to step up and take their fitness to the next level.

During a session about health and well-being I conducted at a law firm for a group of lawyers I offered seven simple daily actions they may consider implementing into their lives. One of them was to simply walk an extra 1,000 steps per day. I explained this would be a short 10-minute focus each day. One lady came up to me afterwards and said she would commit to that one change.

A couple of months later I came back to that firm to do a follow-up session and the same lady approached me excitedly. She looked different: she was leaner and more energised, her skin was better and she was certainly more enthusiastic. She explained that she had started with doing the extra 1,000 steps per day and started feeling better and more motivated almost immediately. She then increased her step count by 2,000 and then 3,000, to the point where she was easily doing 10,000 steps per day.

But wait; there's more. She felt so good she started jogging three times per week. Then she joined a gym, got a personal trainer and was, at that time, exercising four times per week in addition to her 10,000 steps per day foundation. She was loving life. Now, consequently, her family is healthier and more active and she feels like she is a better mother and wife. It all started with a simple decision to do an additional 1,000 steps per day, which led to her feeling empowered and in control and then cascaded into the motivated, energised and healthy person she had become.

So, as you can see, once the 10,000-step habit is established you may very well feel motivated to explore what else is possible for you. If this is so, the first question you must ask yourself is: 'What do I want and why?' Get clear about what you want to achieve and understand clearly and emotionally why it's important to you. Do you want to be leaner? Do you want to feel better about yourself? Do you want to keep up with your children? Do you want to keep up with your grandchildren? Do you want to reduce pain or rehabilitate? Do you want to improve your posture and functionality? Do you want to compete in some physical competition? Are you training for a sport? Do you just want to push yourself, test your capacity and see what's possible for you?

There are many reasons why you may want to step up your exercise to the next level. Decide upon it, get emotionally attached to it, find the right person who can help with it and get to work. As I've already mentioned, it's not the scope of this book to go through every physical option; rather it's to help you make the best decision for yourself and encourage you to get into action. If all this talk about exercise is stressing you out, then for now just keep doing your ten thousand steps per day and be happy and proud of yourself.

Start with a strong postural foundation

Think about how you want to look, feel and function and start there. I would suggest that if taking the next step with your physical condition is a goal, you must ensure your physical foundation is strong. I'm talking about your posture, flexibility and function. I was recently discussing with a friend who teaches Pilates this idea that just getting people to move their bodies is a great start. She looked at me with a strange look and then politely disagreed. She explained that if they just focused on movement without an awareness of their posture and how their bodies moved, it would potentially lead to injury and frustration.

When I thought about what she said, I had to agree with her. Even if walking is the only source of exercise you may be doing, any misalignment, imbalance or lack of flexibility in the body will be compounded by repeated activity and potentially lead to injury, stiffness and soreness. There are many wonderful ways to make sure the body functions, moves and performs effectively. My suggestion is you take your body in for an alignment and postural modification – we all need it, by the way.

When you get your body moving with ease and grace in the way it was designed to move you will get more enjoyment, better results and faster recovery from your exercise regime. There are some wonderful modalities and practitioners out there who can help with this area. Try Pilates, certain yoga practices, kinesiology, the Alexander technique, guided stretching and any other methods you know of that can help in this area.

Taking it to the next level

Beyond the foundations of exercise I've already discussed, if you want more from your training regime this will take some more time, thought and planning. The first question is the simple one: what do you want? Do you just want to be as lean and fit as you can possibly be? Are you rehabilitating from an injury or medical condition and want to get back to full function? Are you in training for an event? Do you play a sport and need specific conditioning for that pursuit? Do you want to be fit enough to be able to live your life to the fullest, that is, have a successful career, keep up with your kids and make the most out of every opportunity?

The key to the success of any fitness program is your reason 'why?' Without a strong reason sticking to it will be more difficult, especially when the novelty period wears off and discomfort starts to take its place. Again, this book is not meant to be an encyclopaedia of exercise options. Instead, it is to help guide, direct and encourage you in the right direction. So, having said that, if you really want to take your training to the next level there are a few things you should consider.

Set measurable and achievable goals. On the way to being the person you want and having the life of wellness you desire, you need to have specific goals along the way. Goals give you focus and a sense of urgency. Goals keep you accountable. Goals keep you heading in the right direction. They don't need to be overwhelming or outrageous; they just need to be there. What's the first simple, measurable goal you want to achieve and by when? How will you feel when it's a reality?

Set a goal beyond the goal. I have spoken previously about a concept I call the 'Everest principle'. It hypothesises on why many people who successfully reached the summit of the great mountain died on the way down. The principle suggests they set the goal to reach the top of the mountain but not to get back down again. I see this all the time: people set a goal to lose weight or get in shape for an event, then because they haven't set a goal beyond the goal they often head backwards very quickly after the goal has been achieved and the event is over. Do you know what I mean? Having a big picture vision for yourself and a calendar of fitness goals will keep you moving and improving and feeling fabulous forevermore.

Believe you can. You can be fitter, get leaner, run that marathon, get into the senior sporting team, get ripped and rock hard, get that bubble butt, fit into that outfit or anything else you are aspiring to. See it, affirm it and believe it. There's no point starting on a fitness journey without the belief and expectation you can and will achieve the desired outcome.

Get a coach. This can be a personal trainer, mentor or gym instructor. Find someone you like who knows what they're talking about, listens to what you want, can assist you in developing the right plan and is walking their talk and get them to help you. Pay them if you need to and be teachable. In other words, take their advice and act on it whether you like it or agree with it or not.

Don't just join a gym; get professional support. I spent many years in gyms watching the same people coming in week after week for years and never changing. They did the same things the same way and wondered why nothing ever improved. We've all heard it before: insanity is doing the same thing over and over and expecting a different result. There are many 'insane' people out there who think they know it all, and I was one of them. It's a waste of your hard-earned money and your valuable time, and it's crazy to just join a gym and not get yourself professional support and advice.

Find a partner. It's always more motivating and enjoyable and helps to keep you accountable when you exercise with someone who has similar goals. This could be your partner, a friend or family member or anyone you can rely on. Choose someone who will get you going when you need it. Pick someone who you can talk to and share your concerns with. Partner with someone who you like and can have a laugh with. Make it someone who will encourage and push you to be better.

Increase your workload. One of the main reasons why people don't improve is because they do the same weights, same repetitions, same number of sets, same run in the same time, same circuit and same same same! They never

increase the intensity. If getting fitter, stronger, leaner and more flexible is
the goal, you must sensibly and progressively increase your workload. A good
fitness professional will help you with this.

Mix it up. Your body and mind need variety or they will plateau. Add as
much variety into your regime as possible. There is no limit to the different
ways you can increase your cardiovascular fitness, strength and flexibility.
Get a plan and mix it up. I will share my exercise regime later in the chapter.

Enjoy it. You don't have to love exercise; in fact, you don't even have to
like it, but it helps if you do. Find things that will give you some pleasure in
addition to moving and conditioning your body. What sports do you enjoy:
golf, tennis, basketball, netball, football or any of the other many activity
types? Make a game of exercise, set personal goals to strive for, train with
others and get excited about knowing that each step, each rep and each stretch
is moving you closer and closer to optimal well-being. That's something
to enjoy!

Exercise is free. There is a massive misconception that there has to be some
type of financial investment to be lean, fit and healthy. Joining a gym costs
money, getting a personal trainer costs money, buying bikes, treadmills and
other fancy equipment costs money. What doesn't cost a cent is a decision
and a creative mind. Sure, you need a good pair of shoes and some training
gear, but apart from that the only cost is the consequence of not exercising
regularly. Get outside and explore the wide array of possibilities. If the
weather is bad or there's another reason why training outdoors is not an
option, look around inside and explore the wide array of possibilities. I can
tell you, apart from good training shoes I don't spend a cent on exercise. I
just get it done.

Breathing is a good choice. It does much more than just keep you alive. In
the chapter 'Breathe easy' I discussed all the benefits of breathing, so I won't
repeat myself here except to say two things. First, focus on deep, controlled
breathing at all times, particularly while you are exercising. Second, introduce

deliberate breathing to your weekly wellness regime: meditation, yoga or just some focused breathing exercises. I started doing this on a daily basis, and it's made a massive difference to my recovery, stress levels and mindfulness and my life in general.

Rest and recovery. This is just as important as exercise. When you are an obsessed over-trainer like I used to be, you feel like any day off is a wasted opportunity to get fitter, leaner and healthier. I can tell you from bitter experience that without a program of scheduled rest and recovery you will lose fitness, run yourself down, stop responding, gain fat, lose motivation, get injured and eventually give up, break down or die. Maybe the death one is a bit extreme, but over-training is a serious problem. Your growth in fitness, strength and wellness requires that you allow your body time to respond and adapt to training, which can only happen in periods of rest and recovery. Your fitness professional can help you with this.

Develop your plan and stick to it

After many years of full-on training, unforgiving routines, injuries, lessons and wisdom, I'm grateful to have survived to the age of 54. For many years I trained for hours each day, lifting heavy weights and putting myself through torturous cardio sessions. I have to admit I was very fit and I looked good but, boy, was it stressful! I now still train on five or six days per week, however, I train for thirty to 60 minutes only. I rarely lift weights any more; I just do functional body weight-resistance training. I do a range of indoor and outdoor cardio training that I vary between endurance, interval and plyometric (jump training). I have to say, at this stage in my life I'm happier, healthier, fitter and feeling better than I've have ever been. Are you interested to know what I do?

I need to tell you that at this stage in my life my goal is to walk my talk, look and feel as good as I can and stay on the path to live productively beyond 100 years of age. Your goals may not be the same, in which case you may need to do different things to what I'm doing. I want to describe what I currently do so you can see that you don't need a lot of time or money, can find enormous variety, train specifically for your needs and enjoy the process, and get fabulous results.

In addition to my goal of doing at least 12,000 steps every day, I train consistently on five or six days per week. I enjoy my one or two days off and I carefully structure the days I exercise so I am feeling better all the time. I do this by alternating days of cardiovascular exercise with days of resistance training. This allows certain muscles and energy systems to recover on days when I'm training others.

Please note there is nothing special or fancy about what I do. The key is consistency. If you train on five days one week and then one day the next, you won't get into a consistent routine and you will increase the chances it won't last. Decide how many days you *will* commit to exercise each week, then make this non-negotiable and keep doing it until it's your habit. Then, and only then, add extra days progressively if you need or want to, and always allow yourself at least one full day off.

In terms of cardiovascular exercise, I do a range of things that are simple and easy to do. The harder something is to do, to organise or to get to, the less likely you will do it long term. Being 54 and a bit of a sook these days, I train inside when the weather is bad; that's my choice. My cardio options vary widely because I need that. They include:

- Going for a run for 20 to 40 minutes.
- Going to outdoor stairs near where I live and running up and down for 20 to 30 minutes.
- Doing a set circuit/run: run to the stairs and do 40 flights; run to the park and do 80 high step-ups; run to another park and do 160 low step-ups; run to a hill and do eight hill runs; run home. It takes about 30 minutes.
- Doing other circuits that include different combinations of running, stairs, step-ups, jumps, skipping and many other movements.

- Inside, I use a video series called *Insanity* that provides a variety of different indoor fitness and strength circuits ranging from 30 to 60 minutes in duration.

The three other ways I vary this cardiovascular training is by changing the style of training:

- Endurance: where I continuously run or do stairs or a circuit for a set time, amount or distance. I don't love this type of training as much as it gets a bit tedious for me and can take too long.
- Interval: where I work hard for a period of time, rest and then go again. For example, I may run five to 10 flights of stairs at high intensity and then rest for a minute, then repeat it 10 times. Or I might run through a circuit once, rest and repeat it several times. Much of the *Insanity* video training I do is interval based. I enjoy interval training because I work harder for a shorter period of time.
- Plyometric: where I do more jumping, bounding and power-type activities. These are good to throw into a circuit for variety and are particularly good if you need power or acceleration for a sport or career.

My strength training is only limited to my imagination:

- There are strength-training videos in the *Insanity* series.
- I have two parks with playgrounds nearby in which I can do a great upper body workout including chin-ups, dips, push-ups, pull-ups, handstand push-ups and a variety of each.
- For my lower body I can easily do squats, lunges, step-ups, lower back extensions and abdominal work.
- I do body-weight and functional exercise and can increase the load by doing more reps and sets, changing angles and hand and feet positions, and varying the speed of movements.

Can you see how simple establishing an exercise regime is? This is just my regime; there are many other options, many other plans and many other strategies available for you. Decide what you want, get some help setting up a plan, get into action and stick with it no matter how you feel. Then enjoy how you will look and feel as a result.

Putting the pieces in place

For me there is nothing better than looking and feeling great. Call it ego, call it vanity or call it whatever you like, it works for me. I love telling people I'm 54 years old and then watching the look on their face as they try to process that information based on how I look. It gives me a buzz. Now, I'm sure you are not as vain as I am, however, I'm pretty confident that you would like to look, feel and function as best as you can. Would I be right?

Developing and maintaining a positive, effective, progressive and satisfying exercise regime is an empowering thing to do. When you are stronger and fitter, you will be able to do more, be more and have more. It gives you an inner confidence that you can do anything and a feeling of power that you are in control. In my football career, when I was really fit, I felt confident and unstoppable. One year I remember going away over the Christmas and New Year period and neglecting my fitness for a few weeks. When I got back and tried to keep up with the rest of the team, it was gut wrenching, lung busting, soul destroying and embarrassing!

I made a decision that year that I would never again let my fitness level decline. I would stay consistent and conditioned. I have stayed true to that decision and commitment for the last 30-plus years. This is a lifetime plan for me, not just a 'good idea at the time'. Exercise is no longer what I do; it's now who I am. I want to encourage the same for you: take the time, build a sustainable regime, stay focused on the purpose for your life and make loving exercise and fitness who you are.

 Key questions and action steps

1. Are you ready to step up your training program to achieve some bigger things with your strength and fitness?

2. Why would you commit to an exercise regime? How will it help you achieve your purpose in life?

3. How is your foundational strength?

4. Introduce some stretching, yoga, Pilates or other core-strengthening activity into your weekly plan.

5. Find a coach, mentor, personal trainer or instructor who you like, trust and will listen to.

6. If you need to, find someone to partner with and/or keep you accountable to this goal.

7. If you want to get serious or get ripped and rock hard, find a professional who can help you, guide you, mentor you and be there for you.

8. Again, if you need any help or direction in this area email me at andrew@andrewjobling.com.au.

Getting the complete picture

As you know, when you are putting a puzzle together you don't pick up all the pieces, throw them in the air and hope they will magically all fall into place. You create your puzzle one piece at a time.

Have you ever heard of the Magic Eye puzzles? They are the most frustrating yet satisfying puzzles of all. You stare into a two-dimensional puzzle and – if you do it the right way – a three-dimensional image magically appears in front of your eyes. They can be so frustrating because if you don't know the trick the three-dimensional image takes forever to appear. They are also immensely satisfying when you finally get the picture. When you've mastered the method, you will see amazing three-dimensional images time after time after time.

You may have been struggling to see the beautiful three-dimensional image of your own wellness puzzle for many years, possibly because you didn't know the method or you were simply looking for wellness in the wrong places: in a gym, a health food shop or a magazine. What I hope you now have is the complete picture, the simple system and the seven pieces of the wellness puzzle. If you put all of the pieces into the puzzle, your beautiful image of wellness will appear magically in front of you.

It's my wish that after reading this book you will feel excited, encouraged and empowered. It's my desire that you will embrace optimal wellness for yourself and your family and – right now – do what you need to do to start putting all the pieces in place. As I said at the start of the book, if you just put some of the pieces in you will see some of the picture and feel a little better. I hope you make the crazy and fabulous decision to be the best you can be, make the most out of every second of your life and live with passion and purpose by putting each one of the pieces in place. If you do, you will see the full beautiful picture and live the happy, healthy and prosperous life you really want to live.

Is that what you want? Are you ready for action? Are you with me? Are you in control and on top of it, or are you feeling a tad overwhelmed? If being overwhelmed is an emotion you are relating to right now, this chapter is here to help put all this information into a simple and powerful game plan to lead you to optimal well-being. Does that make you feel a little better? I hope so.

The seven pieces in summary

Let's begin the end with a summary of the introduction. Confused? Let's quickly sum up the seven pieces.

Puzzle Piece One: Find your purpose

This is the foundation of wellness. It's your purpose that will drive your focus; your focus will guide your thinking; then your thoughts will create your emotions and your emotions will create a positive physical response then determine the decisions you make and actions you take. Find your purpose and you will immediately remove much of the stress from your life. Identify your purpose and you will automatically start making the decisions that will lead to optimal well-being.

Puzzle Piece Two: Protect your mental and emotional space

What goes into your head through your eyes and ears on a regular basis will have a profound impact on your thinking, emotional state, decisions, actions and consequently your destiny. Choose carefully who you associate with, what you read, what you listen to and what you watch. Make no mistake about it: your well-being depends on it.

Puzzle Piece Three: Breathe easy

The most abundant nutrient on the planet, the one we need most and the one we consume 24 hours, seven days per week, is air. On average we take 18 breaths per minute, which works out to an average of around 26,000 breaths and 13,000 litres (3,034 gallons) of air going into our lungs each and every day. This happens whether we think about or like it or not. Purifying the air in your home will reduce toxins, chemicals and poisons entering your body and help you to actually enjoy the many wellness benefits of breathing.

Puzzle Piece Four: Something is in the water

On average, your body is 60 per cent water. Wow! Like air, water is a crucial and in-demand nutrient for your optimal well-being. Remember that every drop of water that goes in will contribute to each per cent of the 60 that makes up your body weight. Chlorine, chemicals, pollutants, viruses and bacteria that happily reside in your tap water will compromise your water content and your well-being. Purify the water you drink and cook with and rinse food with. The difference you will notice is incredible.

Puzzle Piece Five: The power of whole food

This is a large and often confusing piece of the puzzle, and one that took me seven chapters to cover. If I was to summarise it simply and concisely I would say feed your body regularly with a variety of fresh, natural and organic foods. I would also say that when you understand the impact of the food you eat, both good and bad, you are more likely to make better choices. Read and re-read all of the chapters for Puzzle Piece 5 as often as you need to to understand and believe that 'food is thy medicine and medicine is thy food'.

Puzzle Piece Six: Have faith in what you cannot see

When you believe in something bigger than yourself, when you trust that everything happens for a reason and when you have faith that you are being guided towards your purpose in life, you will be calm, relaxed, passionate and grateful for any and every situation. The power of faith is one of the most ethereal yet potent pieces of the wellness puzzle.

Puzzle Piece Seven: Move your body

Can I be blunt here? Just do it! Stop thinking about it, debating it and making excuses for why you can't and just commit to doing a minimum of 10,000 steps each and every day. Everything else will happen from this simple foundation. Do you want to be lean and fit and be the best you can? Of course you do, so get moving!

Missing pieces?

You may be thinking that I have possibly missed some pieces of the puzzle that you would consider important. I also have thought about that, and what I have concluded is that the pieces I have discussed in this book, once implemented, will automatically help with any other issues you may be experiencing.

The obvious example is sleep. We hear how important sleep is, and I agree. I even considered including sleep as one of the puzzle pieces, but decided against it. When I thought about the things that impact our sleep, I came up with stress, anxiety, respiratory issues, medication or other health conditions. By implementing the seven pieces of the puzzle I believe that any and all issues surrounding sleep will be gone, and deep blissful sleep will result.

The wellness puzzle implementation plan

As always, it's one thing to read, learn, think and talk about being happy and optimally healthy; it's another thing altogether to take action. Nothing happens if nothing happens. Nothing changes if nothing changes. I really hope you've enjoyed reading this book and that it's given you some ideas, information and inspiration. I will, however, have failed if it doesn't move you to take the first step towards creating optimal well-being for yourself and your family.

What follows are simple steps you can take to start implementing and putting each piece of the puzzle in place. I first want to caution you about trying to do too much, too soon, which can often be a recipe for feeling overwhelmed and like a failure. Below is a seven-step process I encourage you to adopt:

- *Step 1:* identify the most important piece of the puzzle that requires your attention to start with.
- *Step 2:* pick no more than five small actions you can begin to implement and start putting those pieces into place.
- *Step 3:* commit to three 21-day periods to turn those actions into fully established habits. The first 21 days will get you moving, the second 21 days will get you stronger and the third 21 days will create the powerful habit. Use the tracking sheet at the end of the chapter or some other accountability practice to keep you on track, particularly through the first 21 days.
- *Step 4:* find someone to partner with, mentor you or help keep you accountable to your plan.
- *Step 5:* start today, not tomorrow or next week.
- *Step 6:* every 63 days, pick another piece (it can be the same one) and then one to five specific actions for that piece you will commit to. Repeat the process every 63 days.
- *Step 7:* keep going until you have put all the pieces in place and you have the optimal well-being you really want.

Important: as simple as this is to do, it's even simpler not to do. You won't experience any short-term consequences of missing a day here and there and you won't think it matters, but believe me: it does! Remember that everything you end up with is the result of what you do on a repeated basis, every day, over time. Taking positive actions every day – whether you feel like it or want to or not – will help you create amazing results and optimal wellness. Making excuses, letting yourself off the hook and justifying why it won't work for you will become a habit that will also give you a result; unfortunately, not the one you want.

Focus on what you want, understand clearly why it's important, get emotional and powerfully attached to that outcome and then you are ready to go!

Below are the seven pieces of the wellness puzzle and underneath each one is a list of simple actions you can take – starting today. *Pick the one piece* you want to start with, *identify the one to five actions* for that piece you will commit to and *follow the seven-step plan* I've outlined above. Enjoy the amazing journey to optimal well-being!

Puzzle Piece One: Find your purpose
Actions:

1. Write a list of the five most important aspects of your life. Every day, read this list and focus on it.
2. Every day make sure that the decisions you make and the things you do are consistent with and aligned with these five things.
3. Imagine time and money were not obstacles. What would you do? Who would you help? Where would you live? Who would you become? Where would you go? What would you learn? Who would you spend your time with? Create a vision board with images, affirmations and photos that represents your perfect life. Look at this board every day and get emotionally attached to it becoming a reality.

4. Spend time thinking about and answering this question: why am I here and what is my purpose? Reflect on this every day and make sure the decisions you make and the things you do are leading you to this purpose.

5. Every day, write a list of 10 things you're grateful for.

6. Read a book that helps in this area for at least 15 minutes every day. I suggest you start with *The Magic of Thinking Big* by David Schwartz, *Live on Purpose Through Pathological Positivity* by Paul H. Jenkins or my books *Dance Until It Rains* and *Kicking On.*

7. Set a one-month, six-month and 12-month goal that moves you closer to your purpose. Every day, write them, focus on them and do something that moves you towards them.

8. Get good at identifying your intuition or gut feeling and start listening. It will lead you towards your purpose.

9. Have the courage to change the things that are not leading you towards your purpose.

10. Love, approve of and be proud of yourself every day and affirm: 'I live a purpose-driven life, I make a difference in the lives of others and am passionate about every day.'

Puzzle Piece Two: Protect your mental and emotional space

Actions:

1. Find a positive mentor to help you with creating optimal well-being and working towards your purpose.

2. Make a list of the people in your life who lift and encourage you and push you to be better. Develop daily contact with one or more of these people.

3. Actively find positive, ambitious and uplifting people, groups and networks and create a daily interaction of some sort.

4. Read for at least 15 minutes each day from a positive, uplifting, personal development book, blog or similar.

5. Significantly reduce your daily reading of newspapers, magazines or anything that perpetuates negative news, gossip or fear-mongering with a possible view of eliminating it totally.

6. Instead of the radio, listen to a positive audio, podcast or interview for at least 30 minutes each day.

7. Every day, watch TV less and read, listen or be positively active more.

8. Write a list of up to 10 statements that affirm what you want in your life and read them out aloud every day. Make sure they are written as personal, positive and present statements. For example: 'I bounce out of bed every day and power through the day full of energy because I love my purpose-driven life.'

9. Each time you are confronted by a negative, critical or toxic person, have the courage to change the subject, ask them to focus on the positives or walk away.

10. Every day, share your dreams, goals and purpose with your mentor or positive people.

Puzzle Piece Three: Breathe easy

Actions:

1. Invest in a high-quality air purification unit for your in-home air and use it every day.

2. Change over the products you are using that have any toxic ingredients or coatings to ones that are more natural, for example, sprays, cleaning products, cookware and so on.

3. Start a daily regime of deep breathing exercises so you can start to reap some of the wonderful benefits of getting lots of pure air into your lungs.

Puzzle Piece Four: Something is in the water

Actions:

1. Invest in a high-quality water purification unit for your in-home water and use it every day.

2. Purify all the water you drink, rinse or cook food in, and brush your teeth with.

3. Drink 500 millilitres to one litre (17 to 34 fluid ounces) of purified water every morning before eating anything to flush toxins out of your body.

4. Your minimum water consumption requirement is calculated by taking your weight in kilograms and dividing it by 30 (or your weight in pounds and dividing it by 66). For example, if you weigh 60 kilograms (137 pounds) you should be drinking a minimum of two litres (67 fluid ounces) per day. If that is an overwhelming amount of water for you, start with just an extra two glasses per day and build up from there.

Puzzle Piece Five: The power of whole food

Actions:

1. Eat a natural and healthy breakfast within 10 to 15 minutes of getting out of bed each day.

2. Eat a natural snack with protein every 60 to 90 minutes to keep the metabolic fire burning.

3. Replace some or all of your processed carbohydrates (bread, rice, pasta, biscuits, crackers and so on) with natural fruits, vegetables and whole grains and add a natural and organic multivitamin/mineral supplement.

4. Increase your daily intake of omega-3 fats through eating more deep sea cold water fatty fish and introduce a quality omega-3 supplement.

5. Add a food each day to increase your healthy gut bacteria, including yoghurt, fermented foods, omega-3 and probiotics.

6. Eat certified organically produced foods as much as possible; they have less toxins and chemicals and more nutrient content.

7. Increase your daily consumption of foods that are higher in anti-oxidants and take a natural organic anti-oxidant food supplement.

8. Introduce a natural and organic form of *Rhodiola rosea* into your daily regime to regulate cortisol.

9. Spend 10 to 15 minutes three times per week allowing sun exposure on your bare skin to increase the vitamin D in your body.

10. Enjoy all food indulgences in moderation. If you feel out of control with your eating, please, for your sake, ask for help.

Puzzle Piece Six: Have faith in what you cannot see

Actions:

1. Dedicate five to 15 minutes each day to sitting quietly, breathing deeply, quietening your mind and having faith that everything is okay.

2. Have the courage to read a book, listen to an audio or talk to someone each day to explore the possibility of a higher power that you can have faith in.

3. Practise the *law of growth* each day. Identify the lesson, the test or the opportunity for growth out of every seemingly undesirable happening.

4. Practise the *law of attraction* each day. Be conscious of what you say, think and do each day as if you believed that everything you put out will come back to you.

5. Practise the *law of perspective* each day. Identify the good in at least one challenging situation you face each day.

6. Practise the *law of choice* each day. Trade a negative thought or emotion for a positive one at least once every day.

7. Practise the *law of the path* each day. Check in to make sure each decision you make and action you take is putting you on a path that is heading in the direction that will lead to your desired destination.

8. Practise the *law of intuition* each day. Be aware of that gut feeling on a daily basis and try going with it, rather than over-riding it.

9. Trust yourself every day; you are good enough.

10. Affirm to yourself each day: 'I have faith in what I cannot see and I know I am on the path to achieving my purpose in life.'

Puzzle Piece Seven: Move your body

Actions:

1. Commit to measuring, recording and completing 10,000 steps each day.

2. If you have a medically certified physical limitation to doing 10,000 steps each day, find an equivalent activity and commit to that every single day.

3. Find a partner to help keep you accountable and to walk or exercise with you.

4. Include at least one session per week of functional exercise such as stretching, Pilates, yoga and so on.

5. If and when you're ready, add one extra cardiovascular session and one extra strength session per week in addition to your foundational 10,000 steps.

6. If you have any serious fitness goals, invest in a credible professional who can help you design and implement an appropriate plan.

7. Ensure you have at least one day per week of rest and recovery.

Putting the pieces in place

As you know, when you are putting a puzzle together you don't pick up all the pieces, throw them in the air and hope they will magically all fall into place. You take time, study the picture on the box and sift through the pieces to find the next one to slide into place. You create your puzzle one piece at a time. The same approach must be taken as you put together the pieces of your wellness puzzle and create the picture on the box: a happy, purpose-driven and optimally healthy you.

If you've tried to get yourself in shape with the all-or-nothing approach – exercising every day, trying to eat perfectly and avoiding everything with fat and sugar – you will know that it doesn't work, right? As you've got to this final stage of the book, then I'm guessing creating optimal well-being is important for you. That being the case, let's do this properly. Are you with me? Make it gradual, make it progressive, stay focused on your 'why?' and keep doing what you need to do until you have created positive, powerful and wonderfully healthy habits.

What we're going for here is not just a physical change, but a chemical change. A chemical change is one that happens inside of you: in your heart, your soul and your mind. It's a change that takes time and will lead to the physical result you want, permanently. It will get you off the roller coaster forever. How does that sound?

As you read through each puzzle piece and the list of actions, don't get overwhelmed; be guided by your intuition. There are a lot of things you can change, but start by choosing the puzzle piece that resonates with you the most. Then, as you scan the list of actions, your intuition will direct you to the ones that you need to begin with.

Choose the number of actions you can maintain for 63 days. If five is too many, choose four. If four is too many, choose three. If you only choose one and stick to it, be proud of yourself and excited that you have started on the path to optimal wellness.

This is now where the rubber meets the road. You've finished this book; well done. Maybe it's the first one like this you've read or maybe it's just another wellness book you've purchased, hoping it will be the one that inspires you to take action. Let me tell you quite categorically that the inspiration is not in this book; it is in you. Act now – it is your time. Be courageous and tap into the power and inspiration that is already inside of you.

Get to work today and start putting the pieces into the puzzle, and in no time at all you will put the picture together. Enjoy the journey, get excited and be proud of yourself as you have finally pieced together your wellness puzzle.

 ## Key questions and action steps

1. Copy and use the tracking sheet below to help you stay on track for your first 63-day campaign.

2. Each day you successfully complete the action, tick the box, be proud of yourself and celebrate because you are a winner.

3. At the end of each successful 21-day cycle, celebrate.

4. At the end of the full 63-day campaign, celebrate and reward yourself with something meaningful.

5. Contact me at any time or request a complimentary 30-minute Skype session if you need help and with any one of the action steps or pieces of the puzzle. Email me at andrew@andrewjobling.com.au or go to andrewjobling.com.au/contact/free-30-minute-skype/.

6. Enjoy your transformation.

Sixty-three day tracking sheet

Action 1 (A1)	
Action 2 (A2)	
Action 3 (A3)	
Action 4 (A4)	
Action 5 (A5)	

First 21 days

Day	1	2	3	4	5	6	7	8	9	10	11	12	13	14	15	16	17	18	19	20	21
A1																					
A2																					
A3																					
A4																					
A5																					

Second 21 days

Day	1	2	3	4	5	6	7	8	9	10	11	12	13	14	15	16	17	18	19	20	21
A1																					
A2																					
A3																					
A4																					
A5																					

Third 21 days

Day	1	2	3	4	5	6	7	8	9	10	11	12	13	14	15	16	17	18	19	20	21
A1																					
A2																					
A3																					
A4																					
A5																					

About the author

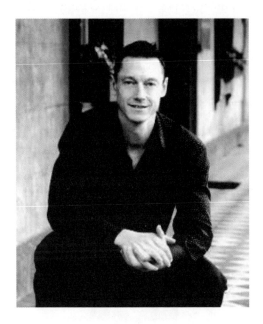

Andrew Jobling is an unlikely athlete, an accidental author, and a true believer that *anything is possible* no matter how improbable or unbelievable it may seem.

Although suffering from middle-child syndrome and lacking physical prowess and refined athletic ability, he did, however, have a clear vision, a burning desire and a willingness to work hard and improve. Consequently, he played senior-level professional football with the St Kilda Football Club for seven years.

With a strong internal desire to help people, he found himself working in the demanding fitness industry. Always ambitious and driven, Andrew worked passionately and tirelessly for eighty to one hundred hours per week in a fifteen-year career as a personal trainer and café owner, until he realised something needed to change. He made a totally illogical and irrational decision that has changed his life and the lives of many people: he decided to write a book.

With no time, training, experience and certainly no clue he 'accidentally' wrote his first two best-selling books, *Eat Chocolate, Drink Alcohol and Be Lean & Healthy* and *Simply Strength*, which rapidly went on to sell over 100,000 copies. This sparked a new purpose and an exciting journey. To date he has written nine books, which have sold in excess of 200,000 copies.

Andrew now spends his time writing, speaking and mentoring to share his powerful message with children, teens and adults – that anything is possible when you follow a considered plan, no matter how unlikely it may seem.